DIAGNOSTIC PROBLEMS IN TUMORS OF ENDOCRINE SYSTEM: SELECTED TOPICS

DIAGNOSTIC PROBLEMS IN TUMOR PATHOLOGY SERIES

Series editors

Arun Chitale, MD (Path)

Diplomate American Board of Pathology (1969)

Surgical Pathologist

Sir HN Hospital, Jaslok Hospital, Surgical Pathology Center

Formerly Professor & Head Department of Pathology Bombay Hospital Institute of Medical Sciences, Mumbai, India

Dhananjay Chitale, MD (Path) DNB

Diplomate American Board of Pathology

Division Head, Molecular Pathology & Genomic Medicine,

Senior Staff Surgical Pathologist

Director, Tissue Biorepostiroy

Assistant Clinical Professor, Wayne State University School of Medicine

Henry Ford Hospital, Detroit, Michigan, USA

Diagnostic Problems in Tumors of Head and Neck: Selected Topics, 1/e
Arun Chitale, Dhananjay Chitale, 2014

Diagnostic Problems in Tumors of Gastrointestinal tract: Selected Topics, 1/e
Arun Chitale, Dhananjay Chitale, 2014

Diagnostic Problems in Tumors of Female Genital Tract: Selected Topics, 1/e
Kedar Deodhar, Arun Chitale, 2014

Diagnostic Problems in Tumors of Central Nervous System: Selected Topics, 1/e
Arun Chitale, 2014

Diagnostic Problems in Tumors of Endocrine system: Selected Topics, 1/e
Arun Chitale, Dhananjay Chitale, 2014

Published by Arun Chitale & Dhananjay Chitale

DIAGNOSTIC PROBLEMS IN TUMORS OF ENDOCRINE SYSTEM: SELECTED TOPICS

Author

Arun Chitale, MD (Path)

Diplomate American Board of Pathology (1969)

Surgical Pathologist

Sir HN Hospital, Jaslok Hospital, Surgical Pathology Center

Formerly Professor & Head Department of Pathology Bombay Hospital Institute of Medical Sciences, Mumbai, India

Dhananjay Chitale, MD (Path) DNB

Diplomate American Board of Pathology

Division Head, Molecular Pathology & Genomic Medicine,

Senior Staff Surgical Pathologist

Director, Tissue Biorepostiroy and IHC core

Assistant Clinical Professor, Wayne State University School of Medicine

Henry Ford Hospital, Detroit, Michigan, USA

Table of Contents

PREFACE:

DIAGNOSTIC PROBLEMS IN SURGICAL PATHOLOGY:

Uncommon presentation of common lesions and rare lesions

Histopathological evaluation is the gold standard in the diagnosis of malignant tumors and chronic diseases of visceral organs like liver, kidney and lungs. Histopathological analysis provides information that helps the clinician to choose the most appropriate treatment modality and assists in prognostication. Notwithstanding the current and future advances in the imaging technology and other innovations, the status of Histopathology will remain unchanged for decades to come.

Whereas Histopathology is the most objective form of investigation, there are many gray areas in arriving at a definitive diagnosis. On many occasions total lack of clinical information leads to avoidable errors in the diagnosis. The surgical pathologist is advised to keep the cases pending until adequate information is available. On the other hand there are numerous problems in histological interpretation even if the entire clinical information is at hand. This occurs because some lesions have inherent morphological ambiguities and no two surgical pathologists may agree on the correct histological diagnosis. One such lesion, for example, is verrucous squamous cell carcinoma of the oro-pharyngeal region or other organs with squamous epithelial lining. The most controversial problem in thyroid disorders is a lesion called follicular variant of papillary carcinoma. In every organ and system, there are sporadic entities, which have debatable criteria of morphological diagnosis. The object of this book is to adequately address problems of uncommon morphologic variations of common lesions and rare difficult lesions with the help of extensive illustrations. There are excellent frequently updated textbooks of surgical pathology, in which all lesions occurring in various sites are described, illustrated and backed by references. However, due to constraints of space, these problematic entities are not extensively illustrated or explained at length. This deficiency is admirably handled in exclusively individual organ pathology monograms. However, this requires the facility of a well-stocked library; most practicing surgical pathologists do not have access to these.

The proposed book is an attempt to address these lesions with multiple illustrations and detailed pertinent text. It is envisaged that the book should be a companion to a standard surgical pathology textbook and this should be accessible just at the fingertips via power of electronic media using internet. The targeted audience includes residents in Anatomic Pathology; young recently qualified pathologists and a large contingent of pathologists attached to medical institutions, in which the volume of surgical specimens is low.

Note on statistical data presented in this eBook:

The senior author (ARC) has been a practicing consultant surgical pathologist for the last 44 years (1969-2013). As a surgical pathologist, he has been associated with 'surgical pathology center' (his own lab). He is also attached to the following hospitals in Mumbai (Bombay): Sir H N Hospital, Bombay Hospital and Jaslok Hospital (all corporate institutions), Bone Registry, Grant Medical College; Cytology department of KEM Hospital.

He has gathered vast amount of neoplastic cases of different organ-systems and the data has been in the form of Tables for different organ systems. The statistical tabulation of tumors has been based on classification of anatomical site and behavior (benign or malignant). This is not purported to be a population based epidemiological data. However, the data likely represents a fair cross sectional distribution and representation of various neoplasms in the population served in Metropolitan Mumbai (Bombay), India.

DISCLAIMER:

Chapter 1: Tumors of Thyroid gland

Thyroid lesions are fairly common world-wide and are frequently encountered in clinical practice. The incidence and prevalence of thyroid diseases vary considerably in different parts of the world. All the diseases of thyroid gland usually result in thyroid enlargement and the term goitre is freely used regardless of the type of underlying disorder.

Except for diagnosis of hyperfunction (hyperthyroidism) and hypofunction (hypothyroidism), clinical diagnosis of various goitres cannot be arrived at without morphological assessment by FNAC or histological study of biopsy, resected nodule or lobectomy. Thyroid nodules (as opposed to diffuse thyroid enlargement) represent a most difficult diagnostic problem.

Non- neoplastic lesions can be caused by colloid nodules, cysts, infectious nodules, lymphocytic or granulomatous nodules, hyperplastic nodules, thyroiditis, and congenital anomalies. Clinically, these are difficult to differentiate from benign (adenoma) or malignant (well differentiated thyroid carcinoma). For example Riedel's thyroiditis, cannot be differentiated from fibrous variant of Hashimoto's thyroiditis or fibrous variant of papillary thyroid carcinoma without histopathologic study.

Fine Needle Aspiration Cytology

This is considered to be the test of choice for the diagnosis of thyroid nodules (1), although in our opinion it is often plagued by inadequacy of the aspirated material and difficulty in separating follicular adenoma from follicular carcinoma and follicular variant of papillary carcinoma. If the yield of cells is satisfactory, the smears are subdivided into benign, malignant and indeterminate grades. In most large series of FNAC cases 70% are benign, 4% malignant, 10% indeterminate and 16% unsatisfactory (2). Papillary, medullary anaplastic and carcinomas, lymphoma in our experience can be usually diagnosed with ease on fine needle aspiration cytology. On the other hand, all follicular lesions including adenomatous nodules in nodular colloid goitre cannot be confidently diagnosed on cytologic study. It is reported that benign cytology (in cases of adequate cell yield) may eliminate as many as 75% of clinically solitary thyroid nodules from the need for further studies or surgery (3).

In our 40 year experience, there were a total of 7190 thyroid diseases of all types, of which 5188 (72%) cases were non-neoplastic in nature; whereas benign and malignant tumors accounted for 2002 cases (28%) (Tables 1.1 & 1.2).

Table 1.1: Non-neoplastic Diseases of Thyroid (n =5188) Author's series (1970-2010)	
Nodular Colloid goitre	3393 (65%)
Benign Cyst (usually colloid)	337 (6.5%)
Thyroglossal Cyst	118 (2.27%)
Hyperplasia (mostly thyrotoxicosis)	460 (8.8%)
Dyshomonogenetic goitre	21 (0.40%)
Hashimoto's thyroiditis	206 (3.97%)
Riedel's thyroiditis	9 (0.17%)
Subacute thyroiditis	4 (0.078
Infective & Non-specific Inflammatory	25 (0.48%)
Non-diagnostic/Non-contributory	615 (11.9%)

Table 1.2: Neoplastic (n = 2002) Author's series (1970-2010)	
Benign (n = 1080)	
Follicular adenoma	1057
Hurthle cell adenoma	10
Atypical adenoma	13
Malignant (n=922)	
Follicular carcinoma	254 (27.5%)
Papillary carcinoma	498 (54%)
Follicular variant	52
Occult sclerosing	4
Tall cell variant	4
Oncocytic variant	2
Mucoepidermoid carcinoma	1
Medullary carcinoma	96 (10.4%)
Poorly differentiated /undifferentiated	33 (3.5%)
Squamous cell carcinoma	12 (1.3%)
Lymphoma	21 (2.28%)
Metastatic	8 (0.86%)

Differentiated carcinoma of Thyroid

Thyroid cancer is the most common form of endocrine malignancy and accounts for the majority of deaths due to endocrine cancers. In the adult population thyroid cancer is more common in females than males with F: M ratio of about 3:1. In patients older than 55 years of age, thyroid nodules in males are more commonly malignant as compared to females. There are a variety of malignant tumors of thyroid as classified histologically. Each entity has distinctive epidemiology, natural history, treatment and prognosis. In the Author's series 81.5% of 922 carcinomas (Table 2) were differentiated carcinomas. In one large series of thyroid carcinomas (4), differentiated thyroid carcinomas accounted for 91% of 1074 cases of thyroid cancers. Among 973 cases of differentiated thyroid cancers, only 34 deaths (3.5%) occurred. On the other hand, among 90 cases of high grade carcinomas (poorly differentiated carcinoma + anaplastic carcinoma + medullary carcinoma) 32 (35%) succumbed to the disease (4).

Follicular Carcinoma

The term follicular carcinoma was used initially because of the microscopic follicular pattern, composed of small follicles with or without luminal colloid. In our experience, follicular carcinomas accounted for 27.5% of all thyroid carcinomas, which is quite high compared to 5%-10% prevalence reported in western countries. This difference is mainly due to the fact that iodine supplements are not incorporated in the diet consumed by Indian subjects. In the industrial world, the incidence of follicular carcinoma is decreasing due to eradication of iodine deficiency and also reclassification of mixed (follicular + papillary) carcinoma and follicular variant of papillary carcinoma as papillary rather than follicular carcinomas (5).

WHO (6) has divided follicular carcinomas into two major categories on the basis of degree of invasiveness: minimally invasive with limited capsular and/or vascular invasion, and widely invasive with widespread infiltration of adjacent thyroid tissue and/or blood vessels. Avanzo et al (7) subdivided follicular carcinoma into three categories on the basis of invasiveness of the tumor:

Minimally invasive: follicular carcinoma with capsular invasion only

Moderately invasive: follicular carcinoma with angioinvasion (with or without capsular invasion) This is synonymous with the term encapsulated angioinvasive follicular carcinoma

Widely invasive: follicular carcinoma with broad area of transcapsular invasion of thyroid and extra thyroid tissue, with or without vascular invasion

Unlike cancers of all other organs in the body, the differentiated thyroid carcinomas do not show nuclear anaplasia, mitotic activity or necrosis. In follicular carcinomas, the diagnosis is based entirely on presence of capsular and/or vascular invasion.

Minimally Invasive follicular carcinoma

Grossly, this tumor resembles a follicular adenoma (Fig. 1.1 A); it is well defined, and most measure >4 cm. These tumors have rather thick capsules compared with the benign counter-part, that is, follicular adenoma.

Microscopic

Histologically, the tumor resembles benign follicular adenoma; however, it is more likely to demonstrate a micro follicular or trabecular pattern. The diagnosis of follicular carcinoma is dependent upon evaluation of tumor-capsule interface.

The diagnosis of minimally invasive follicular carcinoma is made when there is capsular invasion only but the morphological criteria of capsular invasion are somewhat controversial. The capsular invasion is seen as nests of tumor cells penetrating the capsule. In most cases, there are multiple foci of capsular invasion; rarely only a single focus of invasion may be found in a well sampled tumor. In our opinion, mere capsular indentation or location of a tumor island within the substance of the capsule should not to be considered as true capsular invasion. In case of only intracapsular tumor invasion without reactive fibrosis, the evidence is insufficient to diagnose cancer; we use the term atypical follicular adenoma in this situation. The term “atypical follicular adenoma” in the published literature is restricted to a group of encapsulated follicular lesions, which show spontaneous necrosis, infarction, numerous mitoses or unusual cellularity, and which lack any evidence of capsular or vascular invasion. Follow-up studies have shown that these tumors behave in a benign fashion. The penetrating tumor must involve the entire thickness of the capsule and project outside the capsule, not unlike a “mushroom” (Fig. 1.1 B, C, D). Minimally invasive follicular carcinomas have an excellent long-term prognosis and a good patient outcome. The criteria for minimal invasion, although defined in the literature and by the WHO, have been difficult to apply and have led to a great deal of confusion due to the poor reproducibility of the classification and the variable results reported in the literature (42a). Some authors consider presence of subcapsular vascular invasion into thin walled blood vessels as one of the criteria to label the tumor as minimally invasive follicular carcinoma. While others separate this finding into "enacapsulated angioinvasive follicular carcinoma" described below.

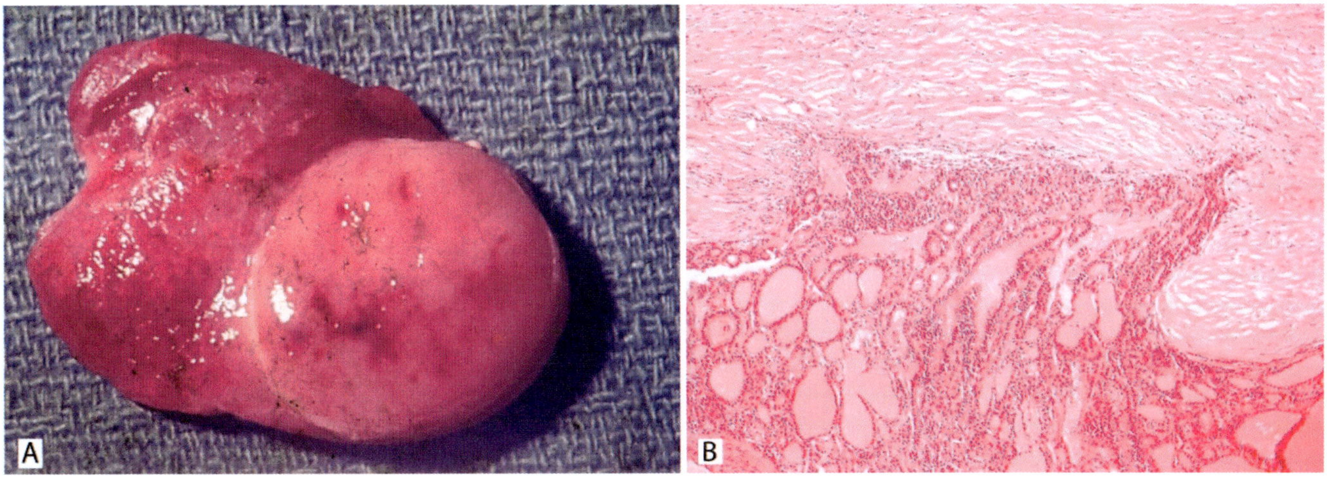

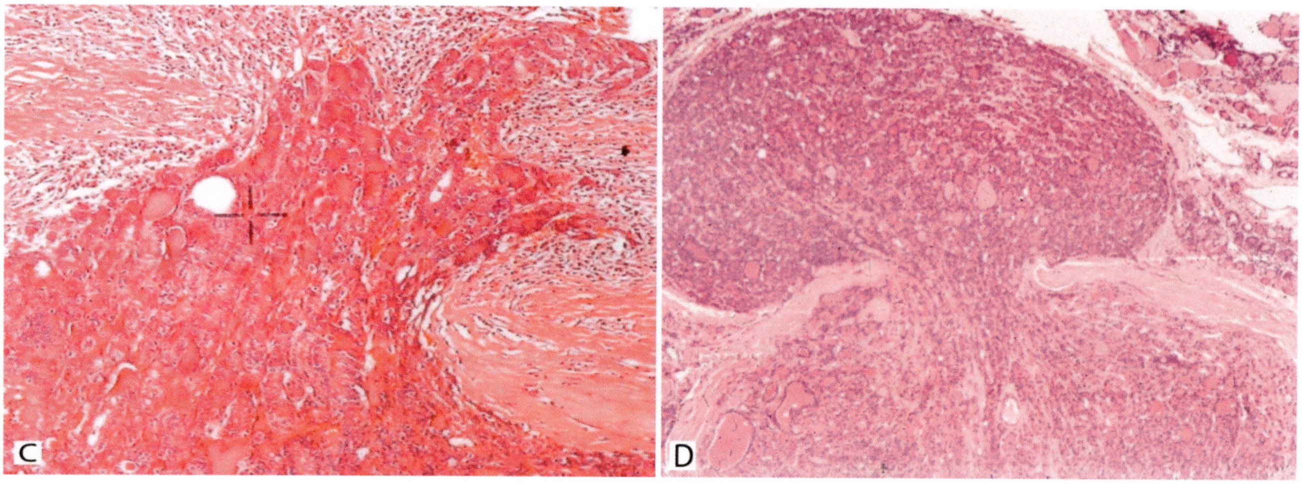

Fig 1.1 Minimally invasive follicular carcinoma: (A) well encapsulated nodule with a slightly bulging cut surface was thought to be an adenoma; (B, C) follicular carcinoma involving entire thickness of the capsule and projecting beyond; (D) tumor invading the capsule and forming a "mushroom" outside the capsule.

Encapsulated Angioinvasive Follicular Carcinoma

Microscopic

This encapsulated tumor (Fig. 1.2 A), characteristically demonstrates invasion into capillaries and thin walled veins, in the capsular and pericapsular region (Fig. 1.2 B, C, D). The following criteria have been proposed as necessary for diagnosis of vascular invasion in thyroid cancer: tumor should form a plug or "polyp" in a subendothelial location and the thrombus should be covered with endothelial cells. The tumor thrombus, thus defined, does not have to be attached to the vessels wall. The requirement for endothelialisation of the tumor island can be waived when the island is adherent to the vessel.

Immunostaining for factor VIII-related antigen and other endothelial markers like CD31 and CD34 is helpful in highlighting the foci of vascular invasion, if necessary (Fig 1.2 E). This group has a significant propensity for clinically malignant behaviour (8).

An immunohistochemical study using immunostains for CD31, CD34 and D2-40 has shown that follicular carcinoma invades veins rather than lymphatics, as D2-40 immunostain is found to be negative for lymphatic endothelial cells (9). It is difficult to understand this phenomenon, particularly since papillary carcinoma usually spreads via lymphatics to cervical nodes.

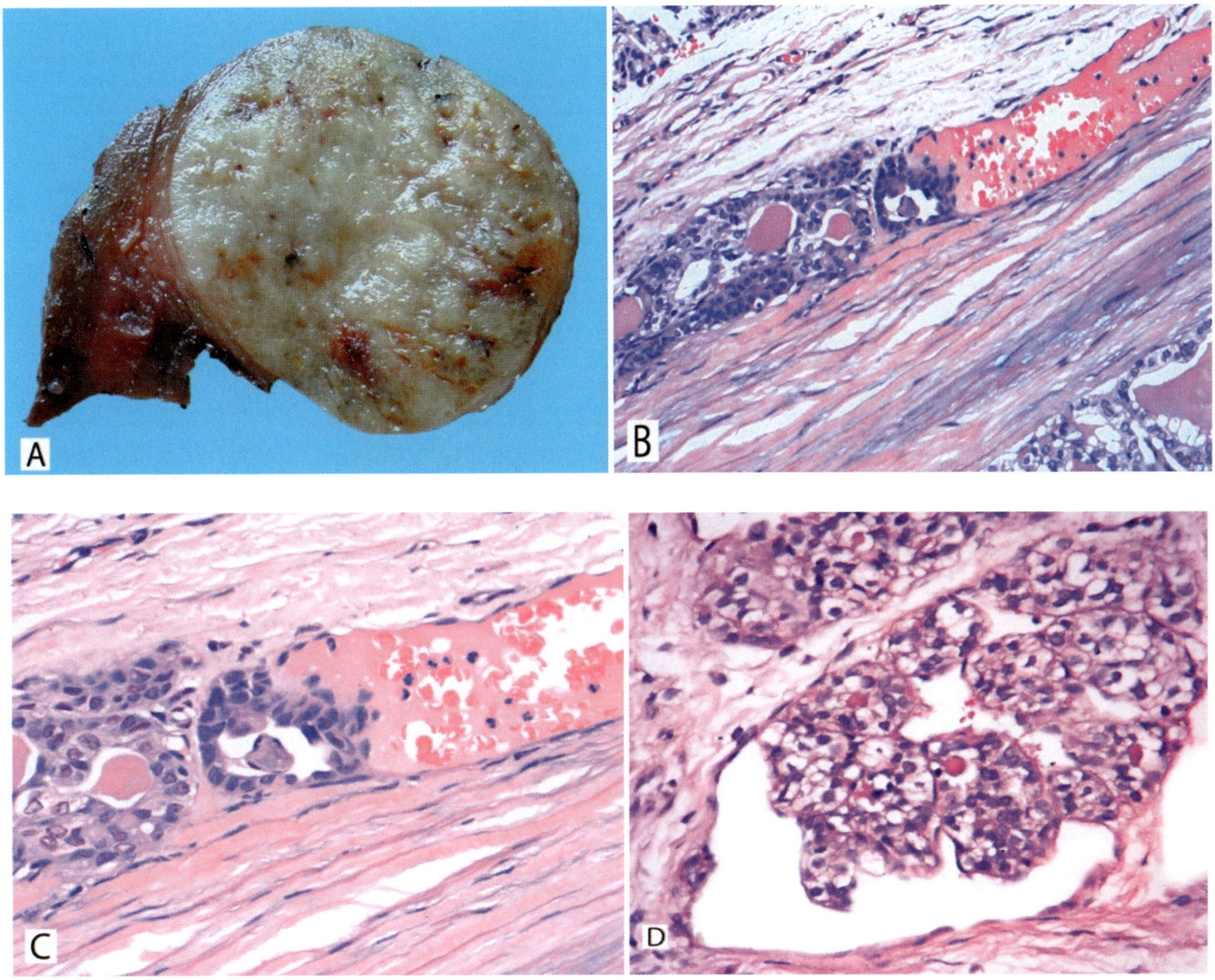
A
B
C
D

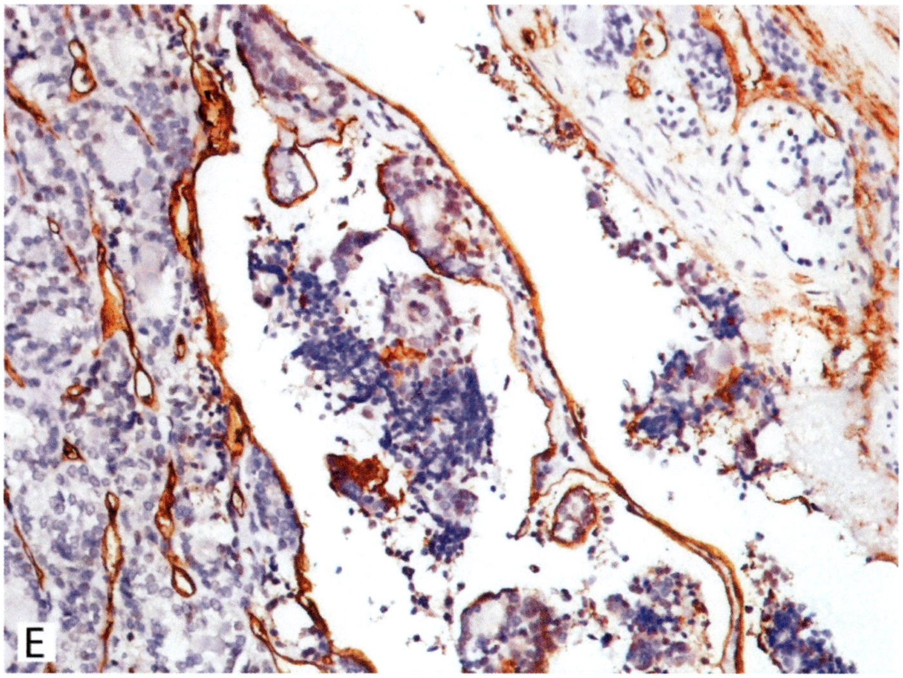

Fig 1.2 Encapsulated angioinvasive follicular carcinoma: (A) encapsulated tumor indistinguishable from follicular adenoma; (B, C) groups of follicles with colloid within thin walled vessels; (D) dilated venule plugged with tumor island (from a different case); (E) fragmented focally adherent tumor islands in a thin walled vessel, endothelial cells positive for CD 34 immunostaining

Widely Invasive Follicular Carcinoma

Widely invasive follicular carcinoma is clinically and surgically recognizable as a cancer; the role of the pathologist is to confirm that it is of follicular origin (10). These lesions grossly spread throughout the gland (Fig. 1.3 A), invade the extra thyroid tissues and often lack complete encapsulation. The most characteristic feature of this tumor is the presence of striking number of vascular tumor emboli and islands of solid nests invading extra thyroid tissue (Fig. 1.3 B, C, D). Widely invasive carcinomas are quite cellular and usually micro follicular or solid trabecular in pattern and may be classified as poorly differentiated/insular carcinomas in some case.

Prognosis

In general, minimally invasive follicular carcinomas have a very low long term mortality of 3% to 5% and survival curves approach those of a normal population matched for age and sex. The mortality of widely invasive carcinoma is high, over 50% of the patients succumbing to the disease (11). These aggressive neoplasms have to be treated by total thyroidectomy, radioactive iodine and suppressive thyroxin.

Table 1.3. Histology & Prognosis of FTC			
Follicular carcinoma subtype	Number of cases	Recurrence	Deaths
Only capsular invasion	45	6(13%)	5 (11%)
Angioinvasion with or without capsular	50	10 (20%)	7(14%)
Widely invasive	24	9(38%)	8(33%)

Modified and adapted from Table 2 in Avanzo A, Treseler P, Iturate PHG, et al Follicular Thyroid Carcinoma: Histology and Prognosis. Cancer 2004; 100:1123-1129

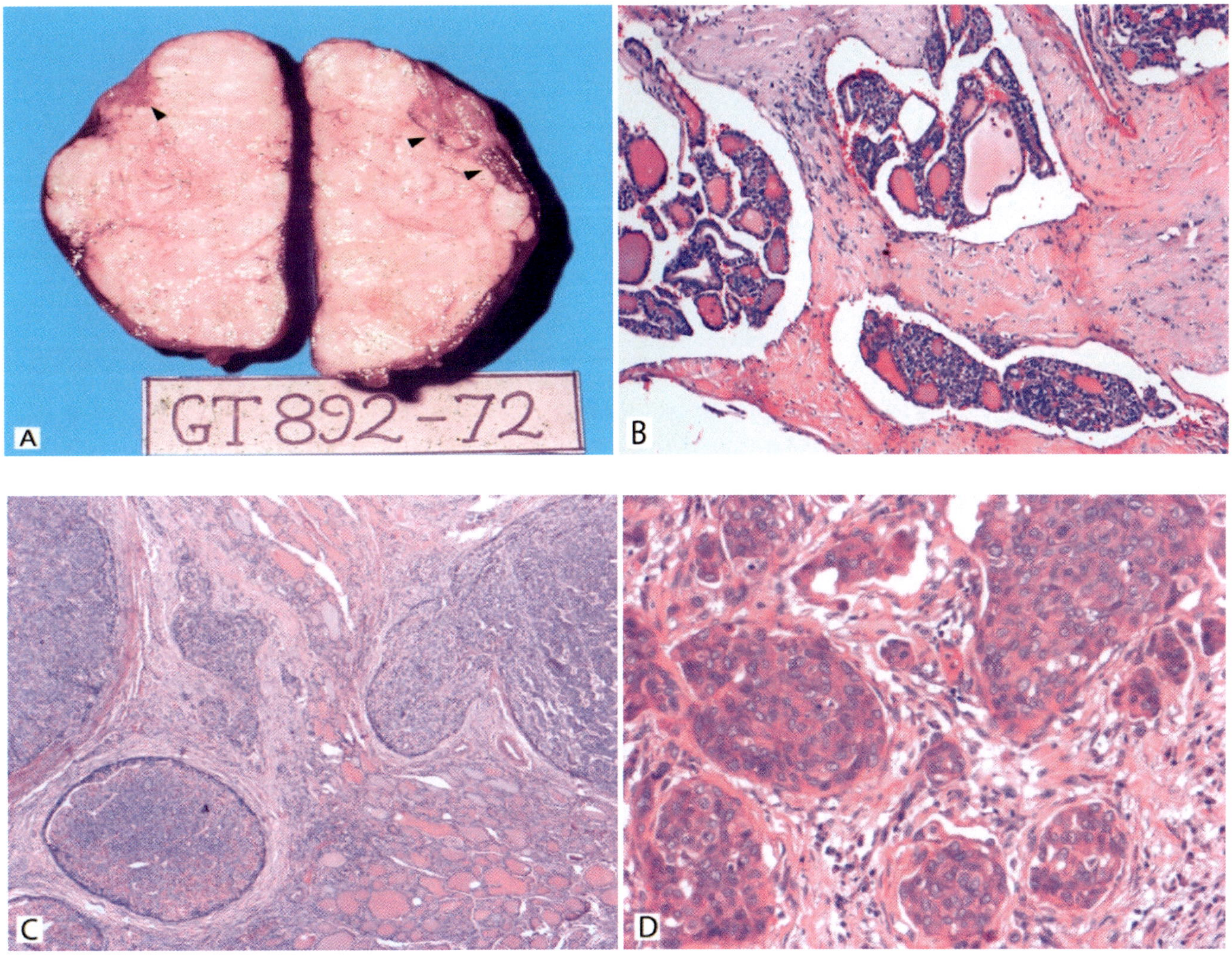

Fig 1.3 Widely invasive follicular carcinoma (A) grossly the tumor has diffusely involved the thyroid lobe with only one area of normal thyroid (arrow heads); (B) note tumor emboli in numerous vessels in the extrathyroid tissue; (C, D) vascular tumor emboli and extrathyroid extension and solid growth pattern.in another case

Hurthle Cell Carcinoma (HCC), Variant of Follicular Thyroid Carcinoma (FTC)

Thyroid follicular cells having large size, abundant granular acidophilic cytoplasm and round nuclei with prominent nucleoli, are termed Hurthle cells. These are also labelled as Ashkenazy cells, oxyphil cells or oncocytic cells. Hurthle cells are seen in varying proportions in adenomatoid nodules and Hashimoto's thyroiditis. Clinically and biologically, Hurthle cell adenoma and carcinoma are identical to follicular adenoma and follicular carcinoma.

Grossly, the tumor is an oval encapsulated adenoma and shows typical mahogany brown colour on sectioned surface (Fig. 1.4 A).

Microscopic Features

The tumor cells are quite large with abundant granular acidophilic cytoplasm and rounded nuclei with prominent nucleoli (Fig 1. 4 B, Fig 1.5 A). Hurthle cell carcinomas exhibit follicular, solid or trabecular pattern, and capsular and/or vascular invasion, similar to that in follicular carcinoma Nuclear pleomorphism without significant mitotic activity or necrosis is often seen in Hurthle cell tumors (Fig 1.5 B, C, D).

Immunohistochemistry

Both FTC and variants express thyroglobulin and TTF1; the results are helpful in differentiation of follicular carcinomas from any other type of malignant epithelial tumors. A series of 23 cases of HCC were analysed immunohistochemically for thyroglobulin, CEA and for immunoreactivity with antibody to p21 H-RAS oncogene product. The results indicated that Hurthle cell tumors produce thyroglobulin and express both CEA and p21, whereas adjacent normal thyroid tissue showed weak to absent immunoreactivity for p21 -H-RAS oncogene product (12).

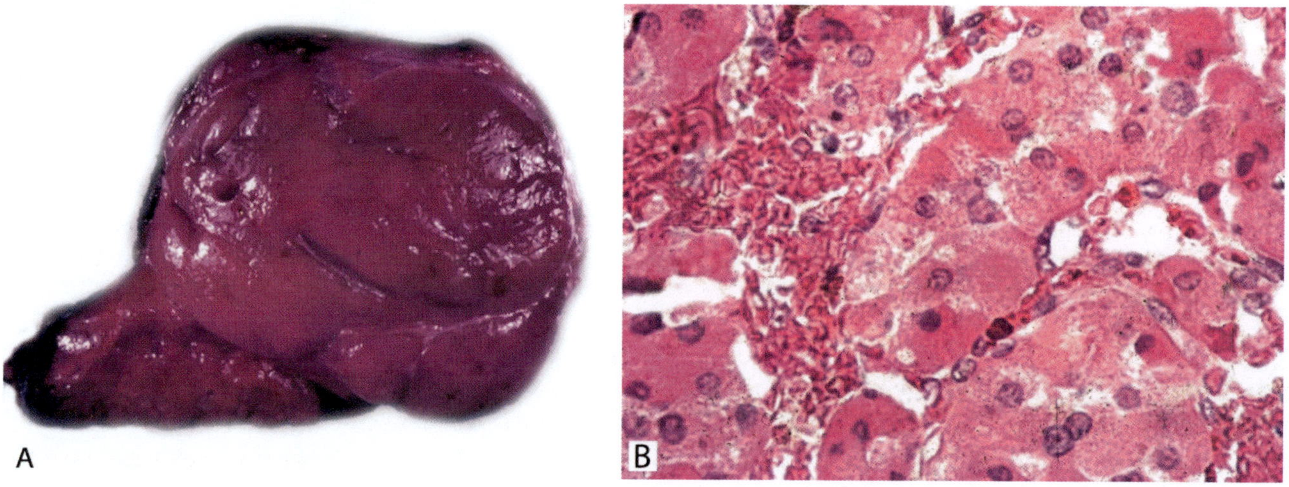

Fig 1.4 Hurthle cell tumor: (A) Typical mahogany coloured thyroid adenoma with no capsular or vascular invasion; (B) large acidophilic cells with uniform nuclei and nucleoli

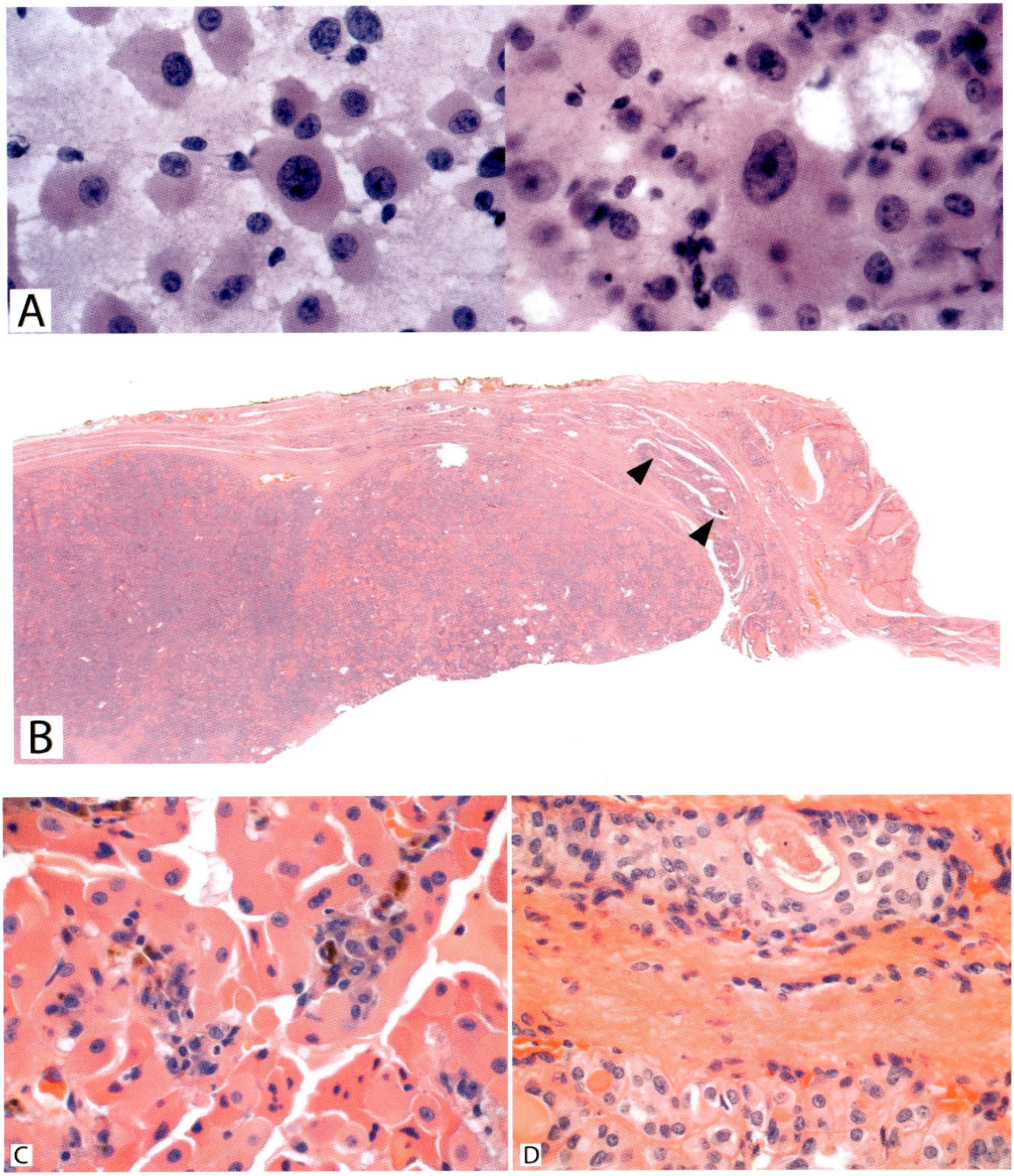
A
B
C
D

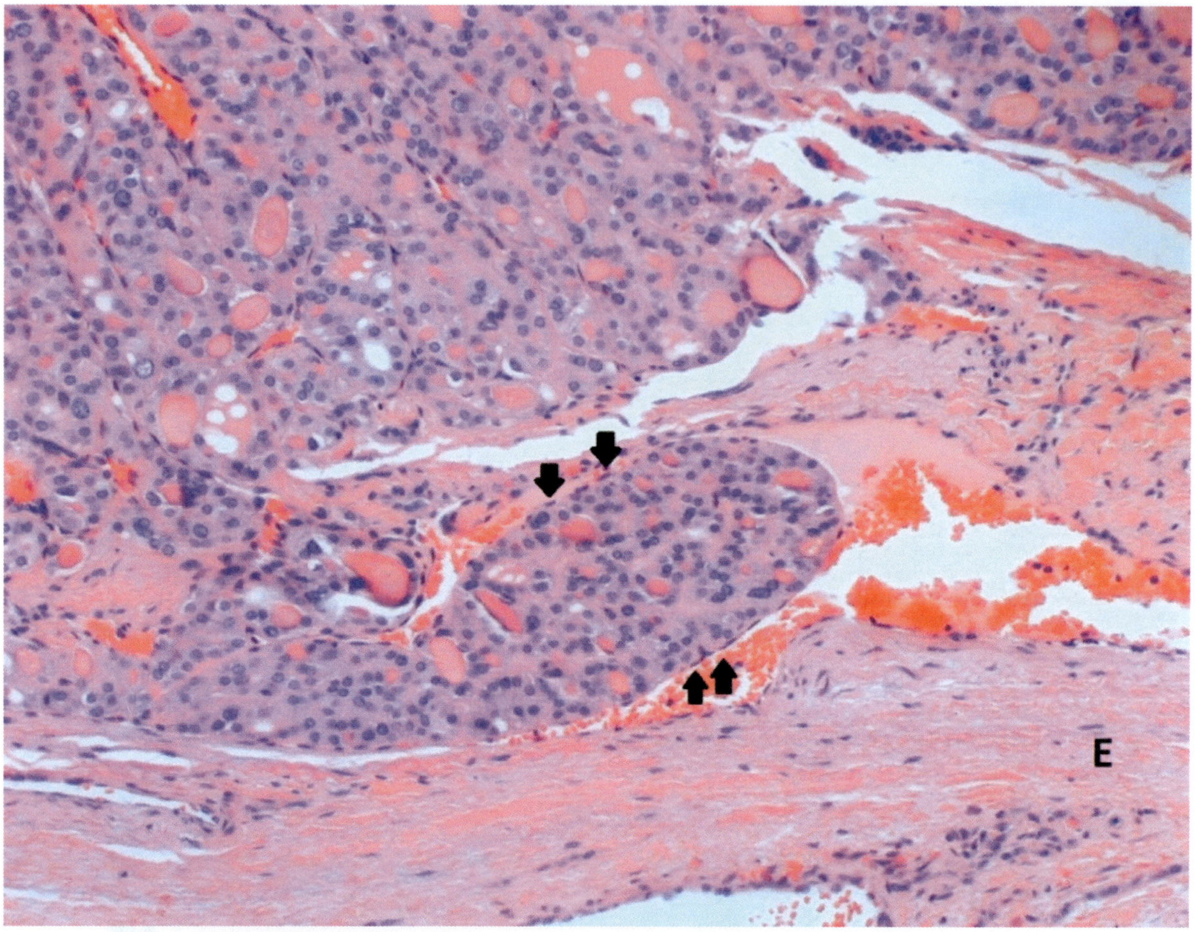

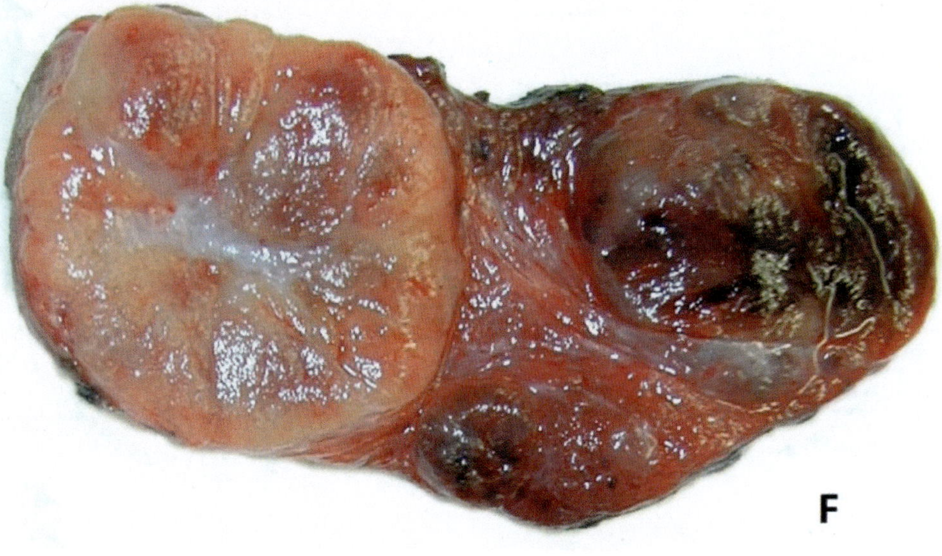

Fig 1.5 Encapsulated angioinvasive Hurthle cell carcinoma: (A) aspirated tumor cells show some degree of pleomorphism but no mitotic activity and were reported benign; (B) scanner view of encapsulated Hurthle cell tumor with extra capsular vascular invasion (arrowheads); (C) the tumor cells arranged in trabeculae and appear benign; of a large compact island of neoplastic cells invading a thick fibroys capsule. (E) Vascular invasion in the small subcapsular veins (F) Gross photograph of brown thyroid nodule with central scar arising in nodular goiter

Biological Behavior of HCC

WHO classification incorporates this neoplasm as merely a variant of follicular neoplasms, others view it as a more aggressive type of tumor in terms of biological behaviour. In a clinicopathologic study of 153 cases of Hurthle cell tumors, 90 (58.8%) were morphologically classified as benign, 35 (22.8%) as indeterminate, and 28 (18.3%) as malignant (13). All the tumors classified histologically as benign or indeterminate behaved in a clinically benign fashion. Of the 28 classified histologically as malignant, 20 (71%) had clinically malignant behaviour. Ten tumors (representing 35.7% of the cases in the malignant category) recurred in the thyroid or in the soft tissue of the neck. Metastases developed in I8 patients: in cervical lymph nodes (seven cases), mediastinal lymph nodes (two cases), lung (eight cases), bone (four cases), central nervous system (four cases), liver (one case), adrenal gland (one case), and small bowel (one case). It was concluded that Hurthle cell carcinoma emerges as a highly aggressive neoplasm. It is of a similar degree to that of insular carcinoma or medullary carcinoma, and apparently higher than for conventional follicular carcinoma. This view expressed by Carcanju et al (13) has been contested by others.

In a comparative study of follicular carcinoma and HCC, it was found that the similarities between HCC and follicular carcinoma greatly outweigh the differences and that it was not found to be aggressive when the cases were stratified according to extent of tumor invasion and compared. It was concluded that HCC is most appropriately considered as a variant of follicular carcinoma (14)

Poorly Differentiated Thyroid Carcinoma (PDTC) & Anaplastic Thyroid Carcinoma (ATC)

PDTC and ATC comprise a small subset of thyroid tumors that are associated with poor prognosis and account for a significant proportion of morbidity and mortality related to thyroid cancer. Both PDTC and ATC display aggressive behavior with increased loco-regional and distant disease. In most cases, patients are older and have large bulky locally advanced tumors.

Poorly Differentiated Thyroid Carcinoma (PDTC)

Synonyms: Solid type of follicular carcinoma, grade III papillary carcinoma, trabecular carcinoma, insular carcinoma etc.

PDTC occupies a position, intermediate between differentiated (follicular and papillary) thyroid carcinoma and anaplastic thyroid carcinoma (ATC). PDTC has been identified as a distinct entity on the basis of the presence of nonglandular components with solid, trabecular or scirrhous type growth patterns (15). PDTC may represent intermediate entities in the progression of WDTC to ATC.

Insular Thyroid Carcinoma

Insular thyroid carcinoma (ITC) is the best characterized group of PDCTs. It was described as a tumor characterized by distinct nesting pattern, small follicular lumina with cribriform pattern, small size and uniformity of the tumor cells, necrosis, and focal perithelial cell arrangement. The striking nesting pattern of the uniformly small cells resembles that seen in carcinoid and pancreatic endocrine tumors and this pattern has been referred to as "insular" by Carcangiu et al (16).

Gross

The tumor is solid, greyish-white and shows multiple foci of necrosis.

Microscopic (Fig 1.6 A-D, Fig 1.7 A-D)

Apart from insular pattern, solid and trabecular patterns are consistently found in PDTC. The diagnosis of PDTC relies on the identification of these patterns together with an infiltrative typa of growth, necrosis, mitoses and vascular invasion. Different diagnostic criteria have been employed by different investigators, resulting in confusion among pathologists and clinicians. A consensus meeting of a panel of experts in thyroid pathology was held in Turin, Italy and uniform diagnostic criteria were evolved, which are as follows: (1) presence of solid/trabecular/insular pattern of growth; (2) absence of conventional nuclear features of papillary carcinoma; and (3) presence of at least one of the following features: convoluted nuclei; mitotic activity of 3 or more per 10 HPF; and tumor necrosis (17).

Apart from aggressive histological features, some cases of PDTC contain variable elements of follicular and/or papillary differentiation. In a large series of 303 cases of thyroid carcinoma, 102 cases were diagnosed as poorly differentiated adenocarcinomas (18). These were divided into two groups: focal-poorly differentiated (<10%) and diffuse-poorly differentiated (>10%) carcinoma according to the extent of the poorly differentiated component. It was shown that presence of as low as 10% poorly differentiated carcinoma component was associated with extrathyroid invasion, lymph node and distant metastases at diagnosis (19).

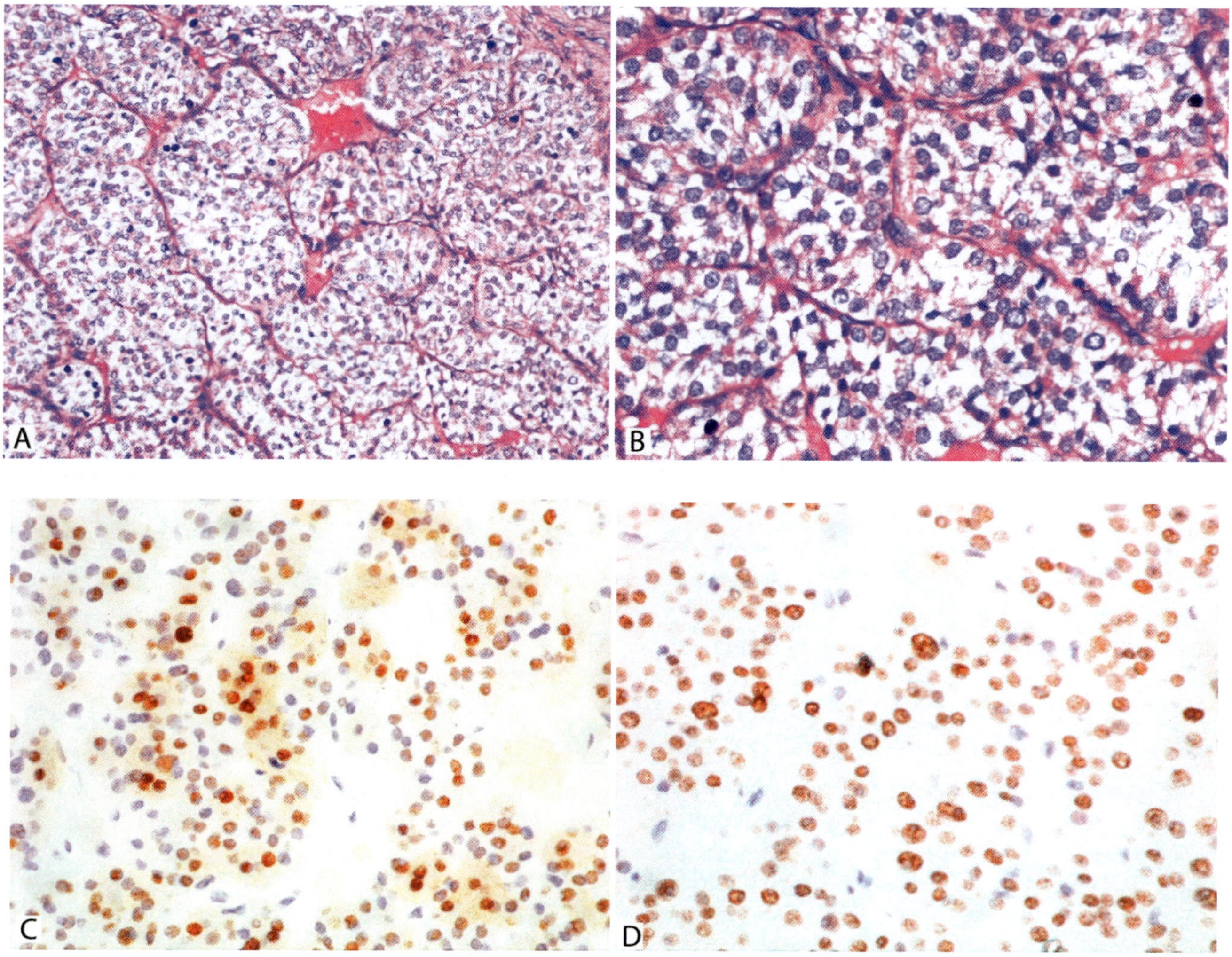

Fig 1.6 PDTC: (A, B) Insular pattern; (C) strong nuclear positivity for TTF1; (D) strong positive MIB1 nuclear reactivity in many cells (high proliferation index)

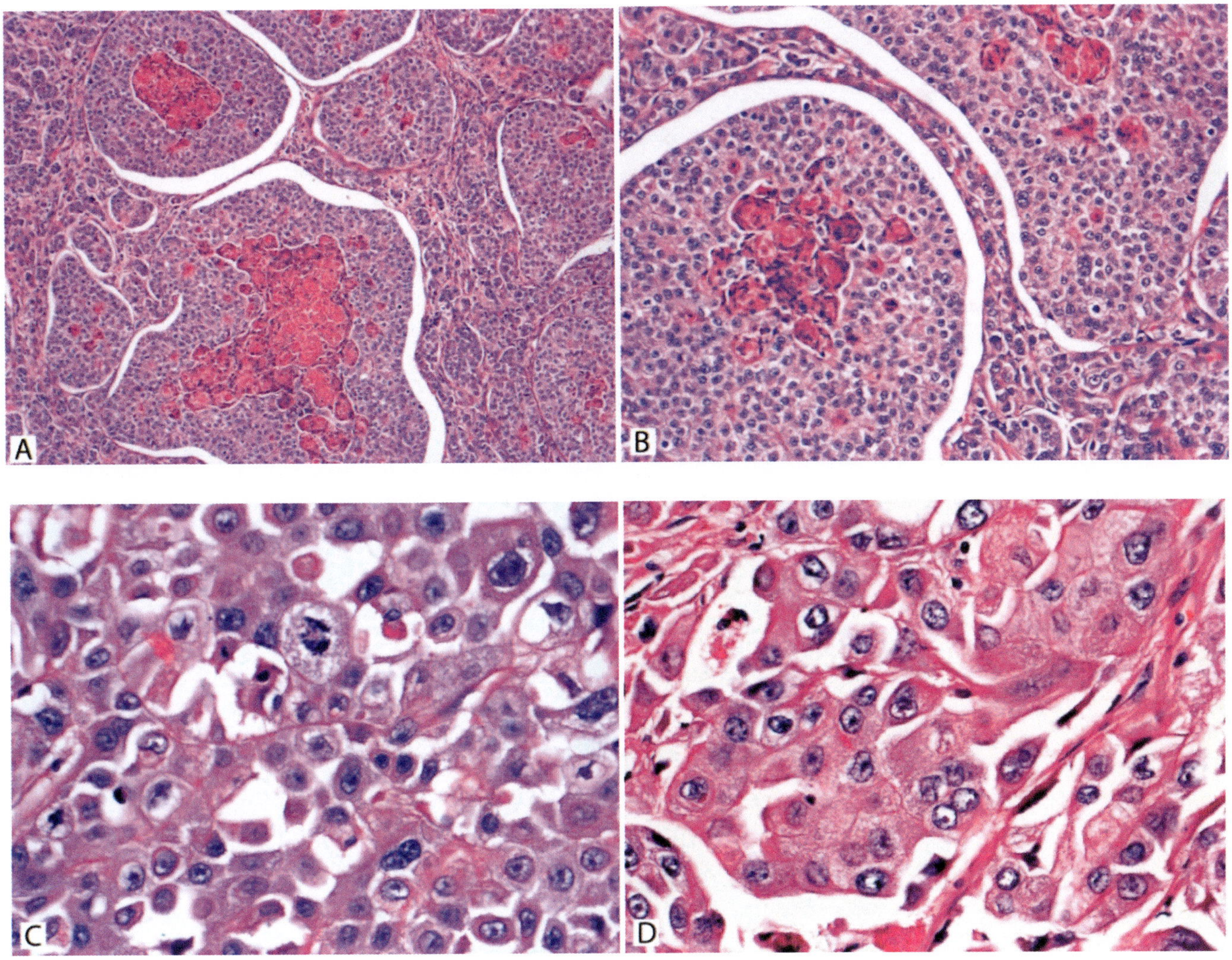

Fig 1.7 Another case of PDTC: (A, B) insular pattern; (C) marked nuclear anaplasia; (D) squamous change

Immunohistochemistry

It has been confirmed that PDTC is of follicular cell origin by staining positive for thyroglobulin (TG) and thyroid transcription factor (TTF 1) (Fig. 1.6 C). The Ki 67 proliferation index is very high (Fig 1.6 D) in this case of PDTC. However, anaplastic carcinoma (ATC) does not stain positive for TG. Immunohistochemical staining for p53 mutation has shown that well differentiated thyroid carcinoma is not stained. Expression of BcL-2 and p53 was investigated by immunohistochemistry for 19 cases of PDTC and 22 cases of ATC. P53 was expressed in 52% of cases of PDTC and 54% of cases of ATC. However, the pattern of distribution of p53 immunoreactive cells was different, being restricted to areas of active infiltrative growth in PDTC and involving almost all cells in ATC (20)

Prognosis

The mean five-year survival rate is about 50% for PDTC in most series, and the majority of patients die in the first 3 years after diagnosis and few survive >5 years.

Undifferentiated Thyroid Carcinoma (ATC)

The term undifferentiated thyroid carcinoma (UTC) is more appropriate than anaplastic carcinoma because it does not make follicles, papillae or trabeculae and most commonly presents as a giant cell and/or spindle cell sarcomatoid morphology. This tumor is called carcinoma (not sarcoma) because almost all cases strongly express cytokeratins.

UTC is the most aggressive human tumor and most patients die within 1 year of diagnosis. It commonly occurs in elderly subjects, usually females and constitutes over 5% of all thyroid malignancies (21). A clinicopathologic data on 124 patients of undifferentiated carcinoma (4.24% of a total of 2921 thyroid carcinomas), treated at the Tata Memorial Hospital in Mumbai, revealed 50% of patients had either long standing goitres, previous thyroid abnormalities or associated differentiated carcinoma (22). Anaplastic transformation may be induced by the administration of radioactive Iodine for treatment of differentiated thyroid carcinoma (21, 22,23). In a clinicopathologic study of 121 cases of undifferentiated carcinoma, 35% had areas of well- differentiated thyroid carcinoma, supporting the hypothesis that undifferentiated carcinomas arise from pre-existing well differentiated thyroid carcinoma (24). In a recent study, Hunt et al examined the molecular mutational profile of tumor suppressor genes in concurrent anaplastic and well-differentiated thyroid carcinoma. The study demonstrated definitive evidence of molecular progression of de-differentiation at the genetic level (25).

Gross

UTC is a very large unencapsulated firm focally necrotic grey white tumor replacing the thyroid glands and exhibiting extensive infiltration in the soft tissues of the neck.

Microscopic

Three histologic patterns are commonly described: spindle cell, giant cell (Fig. 1.8 A-D)) and squamoid. There is no prognostic difference in these patterns. All three variants have numerous mitotic figures, with large areas of necrosis, haemorrhages and vascular invasion. (26) A rare variant of UTC called paucicellular variant shows few malignant cells embedded in a densely sclerotic stroma and this may be mistaken for Riedel's disease.(27)

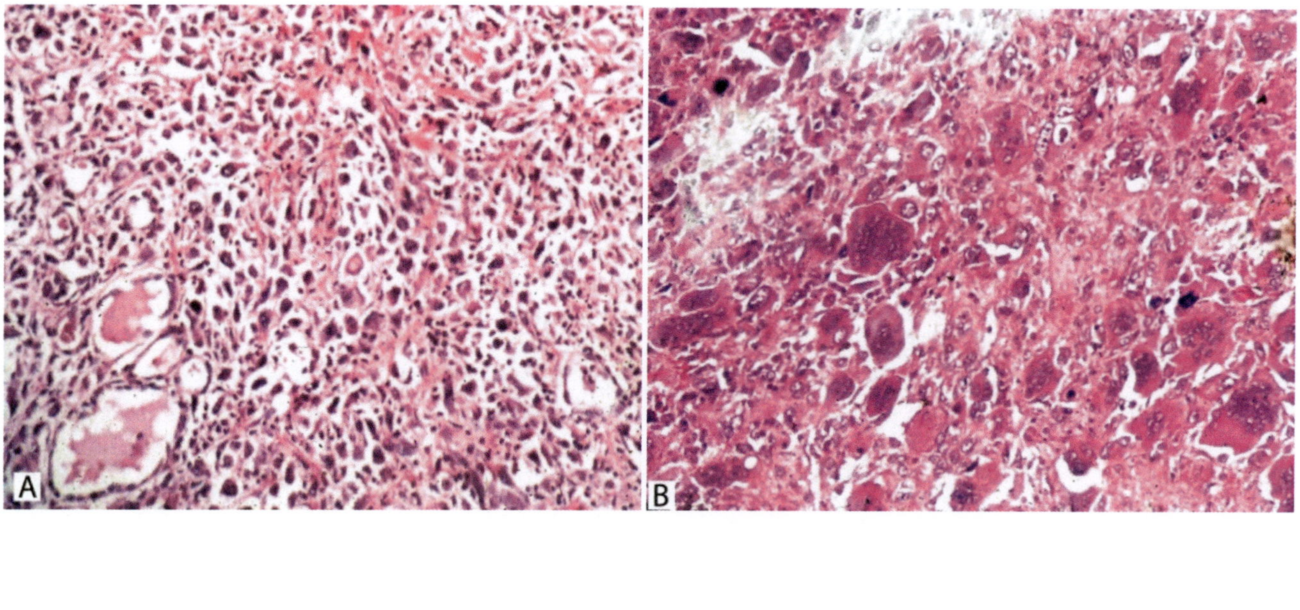

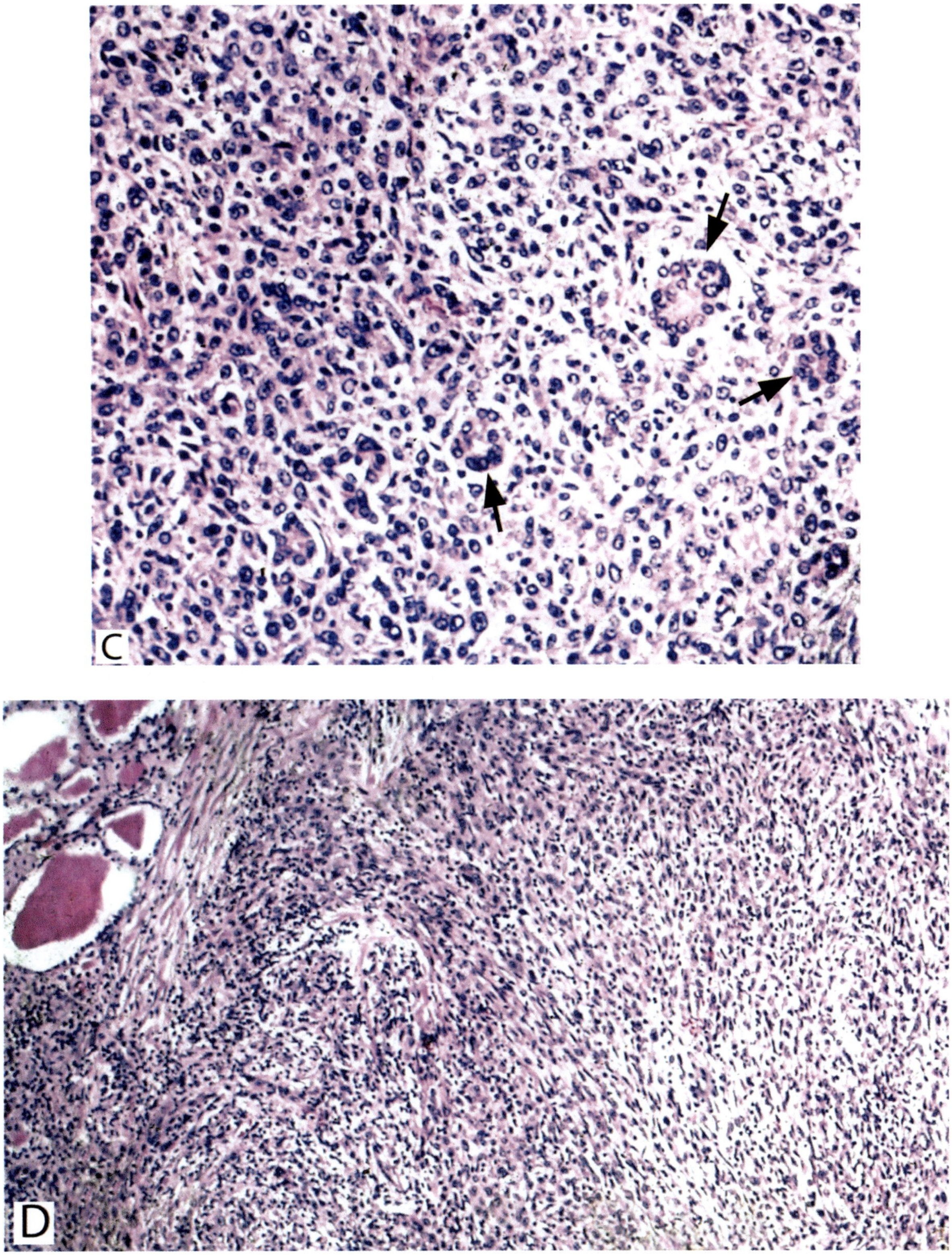

Fig 1.8 undifferentiated (anaplastic) carcinoma: (A, B) predominantly giant cell malignant tumor with osteoclastic type giant cells in (B); (C, D) anaplastic small spindle cell tumor with occasional abortive acinus (arrows) in (C); (D) few benign (normal) host thyroid acini (left upper corner,) in both cases illustrated here thyroglobulin or TTF 1 antigen are not expressed.

Prognosis

The overall five-year survival ranges from 0-14% and the median survival is 2.5-6 months (11a).

Papillary Thyroid Carcinoma (PTC) & Variants

PTC comprises approximately 80%-85% of malignant epithelial tumors of the thyroid in geographic regions where sufficient iodine is present in the diet. It is common in adults (in less than 40 years of age) and is three times more common in women. It is also the most common thyroid malignancy in paediatric population. Follicular and anaplastic carcinomas are common in regions of endemic goiter. A fair number of PTCs develop from a gland harbouring multinodular goiter, chronic thyroiditis and Grave's disease, all of which are common.

Gross

The tumor size can range from less than a centimeter, classified as 'microcarcinoma' to a bulky tumor involving the entire lobe with extension beyond the gland. Intracystic papillary growth formation is not an uncommon finding (Fig.1. 9 A). In some cases, extension of the tumor in the neck is appreciated clinically at the time of presentation. Papillary carcinoma often spreads into lymphatic channels and hence regional lymph node metastasis at presentation is found in significant proportion of patients. Metastatic tumor in the neck nodes can form masses, usually larger than that of the primary in the lobe (Fig. 1.9 B). The metastatic nodal masses may show hemorrhagic cystic change at times (Fig. 1.10)

Microscopic

The conventional TPC shows a papillary growth pattern, the papillae exhibiting delicate central fibrovascular cores with complex branching structure. However, definitive diagnosis is established solely on nuclear features (Fig.1. 9 C, D). The nuclei of PTC are oval shaped and show nuclear chromatin clearing ("Orphan Annie" or ground glass nucleus), nuclear grooves, intranuclear inclusions and small eccentric nucleoli. The distinction between papillary and follicular carcinomas is not as easy as it appears from morphologic standpoint because very few PTCs are exclusively formed of papillae. In the past, the tumor was named as PTC or FTC according to the predominant pattern and the pathologist then used the term mixed carcinoma when the two components were roughly equal (28).

In some cases, the formation of papillae is so sparse that these have to be searched for in a study of multiple sections of the lesion. However, the characteristic nuclear changes can readily differentiate PTC from follicular carcinoma. Psammoma bodies, which appear as round and labelled calcified bodies, are always encountered in PTC with papillary growth pattern. Nearly 45% of PTCs show squamous metaplasia (29).

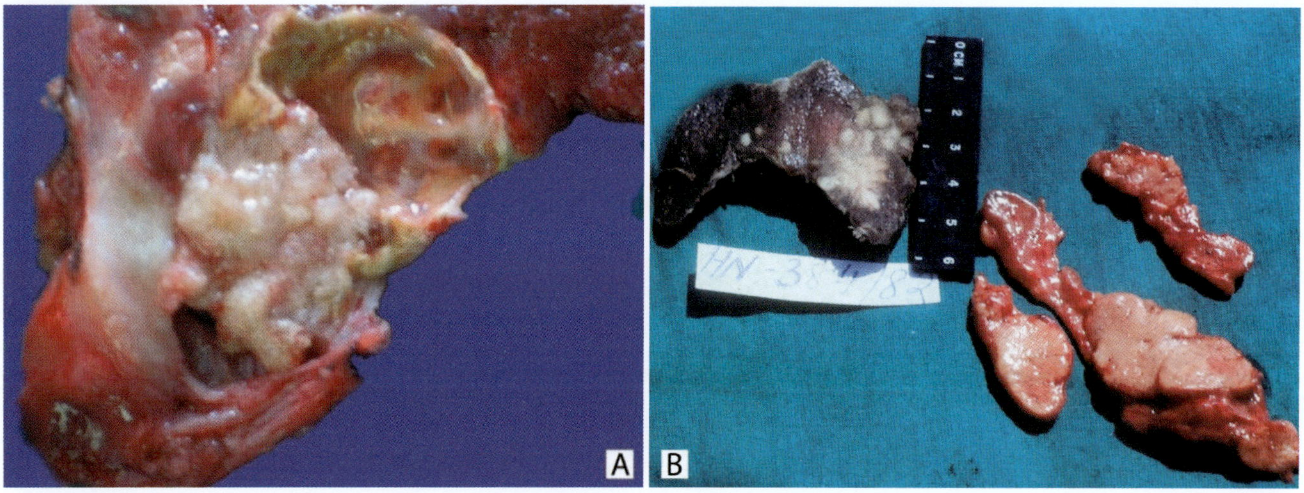

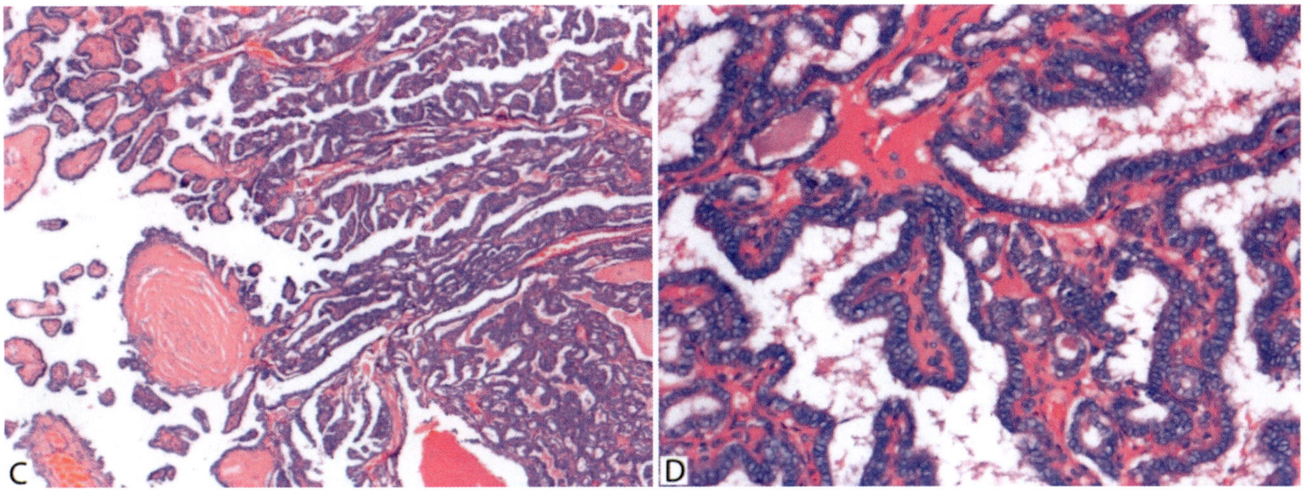

Fig. 9. PTC: (A) gross appearance of cystic papillary carcinoma; (B) a 3 cm solid growth in one lobe with metastases to many cervical nodes; (C, D) complex papillary pattern with delicate supporting vascular strands and nuclei with clear chromatin ("Orphan Annie" nuclei)

PTC always spreads via lymphatics within and outside the thyroid gland and it is believed that multiple isolated foci of the tumor are seen within the gland and represent intrathyroid metastases (30). Lymph node metastasis occurs in 42%-90% of cases of PTC; vascular invasion seen up to 7% of cases and distant metastasis to lung and bones in 5%-7% of cases (31).

Papillary microcarcinoma of thyroid (PMC) variant

The term microcarcinoma should be used for a papillary carcinoma, which measures 1 cm or less in diameter. These lesions are frequently detected as incidental findings at autopsy or in surgical specimens. PMC has been reported in up to 24% of thyroidectomies performed for diseases unrelated to papillary carcinomas (32). They are often multifocal. In patients with clinical thyroid cancer, PMC may represent intrathyroid metastases; they may be the earliest form of future large lesions. The relationship between PMC and clinical papillary thyroid carcinoma (PTC) is not clear. Many cases of PMC first present as lymph node metastasis and the primary is identified after study of surgical specimen. Usually, papillary microcarcinoma behaves in a benign fashion; however, Hazard, Woolner and associates have shown that 23% and 43% of their cases of occult carcinoma, respectively, metastasized to cervical lymph nodes (33, 34). Cervical node metastases from thyroid carcinomas even less than 1 mm in diameter have also been reported (Fig. 1.10). The prognosis of PMC with nodal metastasis is excellent and occurrence of blood borne metastasis is exceptional (35). The prognosis of PMC is good in vast majority of cases but there have been hardly any studies concerning factors predictive of lymph node and distant metastasis. Recently, Min et al have shown that S100A4 expression in papillary microcarcinoma may be valuable in predicting its metastatic potential (36).

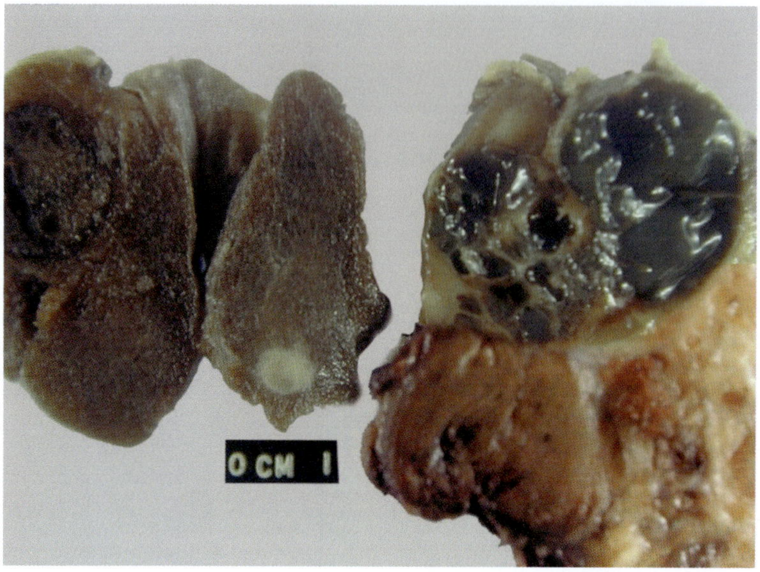

Fig 1.10 Papillary microcarcinoma: 5 mm growth in one lobe with large hemorrhagic tumor deposits in ipsilateral cervical nodes. In this case, the thyroid gland was normal on clinical examination. Note the size of the metastatic disease in nodes.

Follicular Variant of Papillary Thyroid Carcinoma (FVPTC)

FVPTC is the third most common type of papillary thyroid carcinoma following conventional TPC and papillary microcarcinoma (PMC). There has been a constant debate regarding the optimal classification, treatment and prognosis of the FVPTC. The tumor is further subdivided into encapsulated (Fig. 11 A) and non-encapsulated (infiltrative or diffuse), latter reported to be clinically aggressive. It is further separated into tumor with or without capsular/vascular invasion (37). The diagnosis depends entirely on demonstration of nuclear changes (nuclear chromatin clearing, grooves and pseudoinclusions) similar to those in conventional papillary carcinoma (Fig. 1.11 C, D). The case illustrated here, showed capsular invasion and displayed massive lymphadenopathy (Fig. 1.11 B). FVPTC cases clinically present either as a single nodule or can arise against a background of multinodular goitre (Fig. 1.12A, B) (10). FVPTC cases resemble conventional PTC in the biological behavior and nuclear features but in the follicular variant papillae are never seen (38). At the genetic level, FVPTC have been shown to have profiles similar to follicular adenoma / carcinoma. For example, array comparative genomic hybriduzaion (aCGH) analyses have shown patterns of chromosomal aberrations similar to follicular adenona and follicular carcinoma and different from classic PTC. In addition, RAS mutations are common in FVPTC similar to follicular adenona and follicular carcinoma and BRAF mutations and RET gene rearrangements are indeed rare which are common in classic PTC.

Follicular-patterned lesions of thyroid

Follicular variant of papillary thyroid carcinoma (FVPTC) (Fig. 1.11 A, B, C, D)
Follicular variant arising in nodular colloid goitre (Fig. 1.12 A, B)
Follicular adenoma (No capsular or vascular invasion)
Follicular Adenomatous nodule (Figure 1.13)

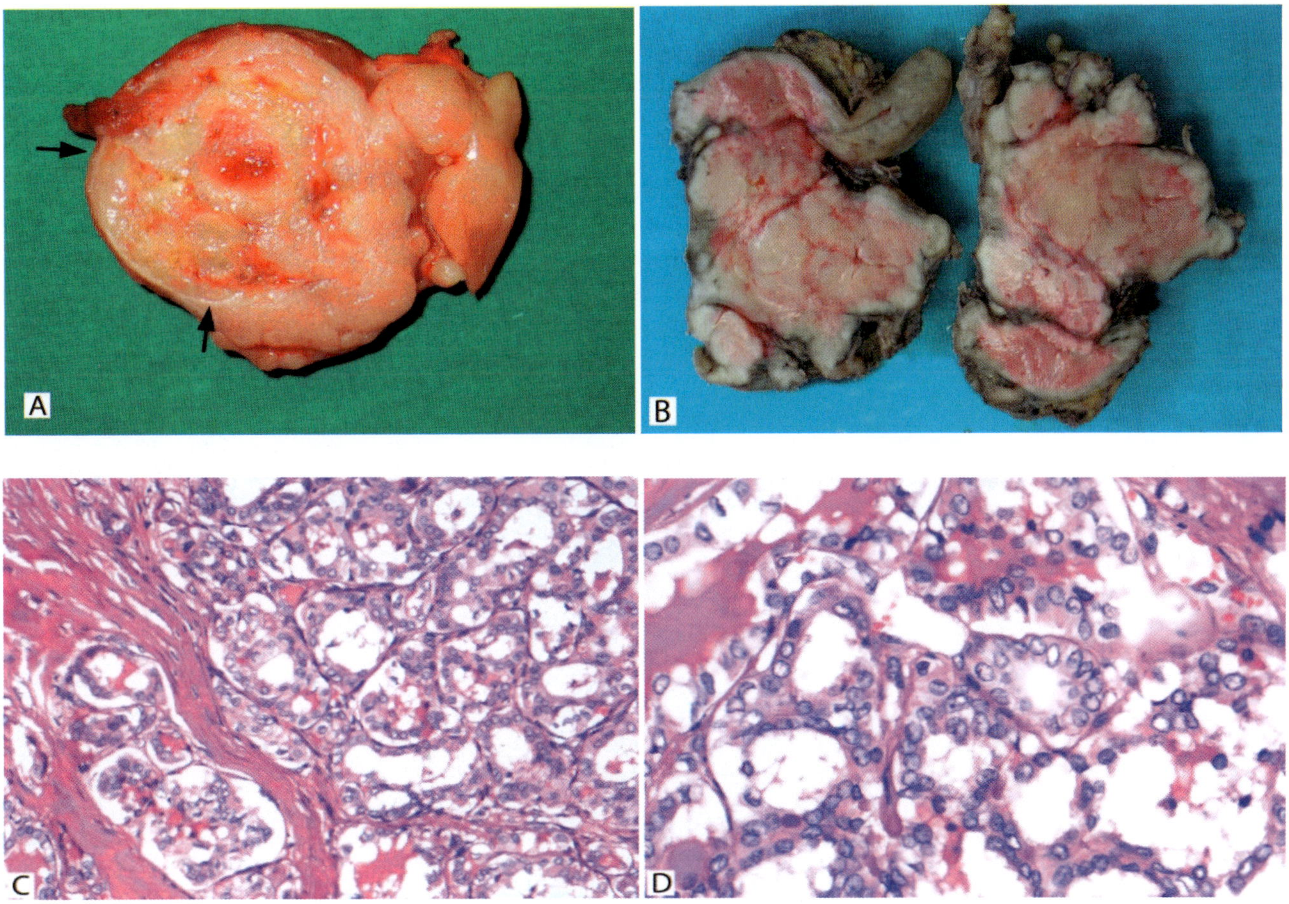

Fig 1.11 FVPTC: (A) partly encapsulated (arrows) spherical mass; (B) massive tumor deposits in bilateral cervical nodes; (C) pure follicular-patterned papillary carcinoma with capsular invasion; (D) close up of (C) to show "Orphan Annie" nuclei

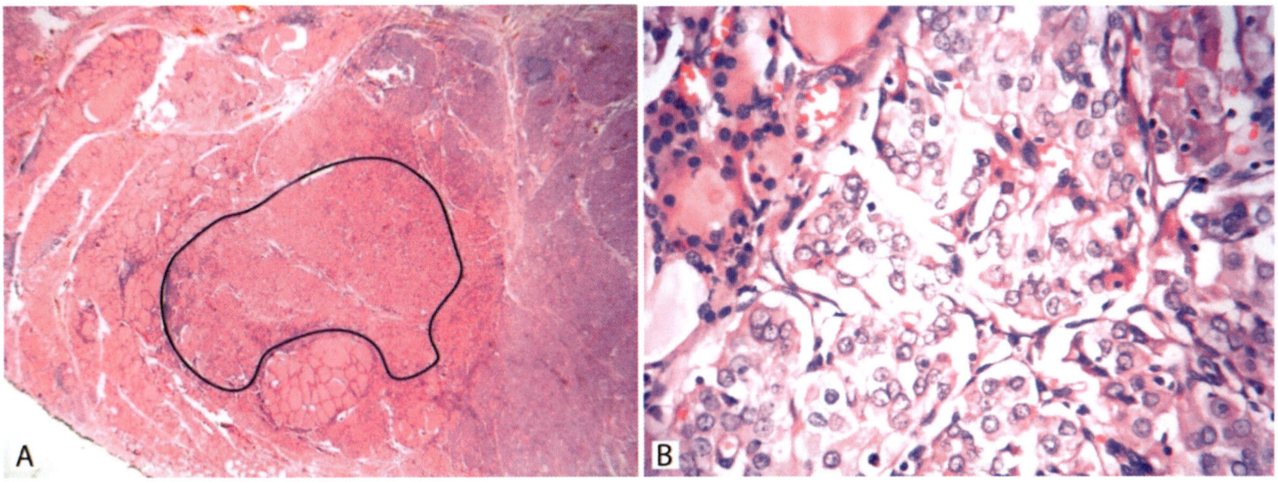

Fig 1.12 Nodular goiter with associated infiltrating FVTPC: (A) scanner view shows a circumscribed more cellular tumor (bracketed) within nodular goitre; (B) follicular pattern and typical nuclear characteristicsare present

Follicular adenomatous nodule

Most of these lesions can be diagnosed with ease. In general, the nuclear features of papillary thyroid carcinomas are one of the most important and reproducible criteria (a gold standard) in the diagnosis of thyroid tumors, and FVPTC can be readily differentiated from other follicular-patterned lesions when they are conspicuous (39). The diagnostic dilemma comes when focal nuclear features of PTC are noted in otherwise nodular goiter or "adenomatoid hyperplasia" without capular or vascular invasion. The diagnosis of such lesions as carcinoma is controversial. When mutiple foci with cytological features of PTC are noted in a follicular-patterned encapsulated thyroid nodule, some authors suggest two ways of interpretations: 1. To tally and report all such foci with PTC nuclear features as multiple foci of micro-PTC arising in a benign nodule (each less than 1 cm) or 2. consider the entire nodule as FVPTC (10). LiVolsi et al use second approach and have shown follicular adenoma or tumors of uncertain malignant potential on the basis of minimal nuclear featurs of PTC later developed lymph node and bone metastasis (8). Follicular adenoma and encapsulated folicular carcinoma can be set apart on the basis of capsular and/or vascular invasion.

A majority of clinically diagnosed single nodules turn out to be part of nodular colloid goiter, which is the end result of many cycles of hyperplasia and involution. In some cases, a hyperplastic or adenomatous nodule shows partial or complete encapsulation and may mimic follicular adenoma (Fig. 1.13). It is postulated that malignant transformation in follicular-patterned lesions of the thyroid involves a sequence of molecular events originating in adenomatoid hyperplasia and leading to carcinoma (10).

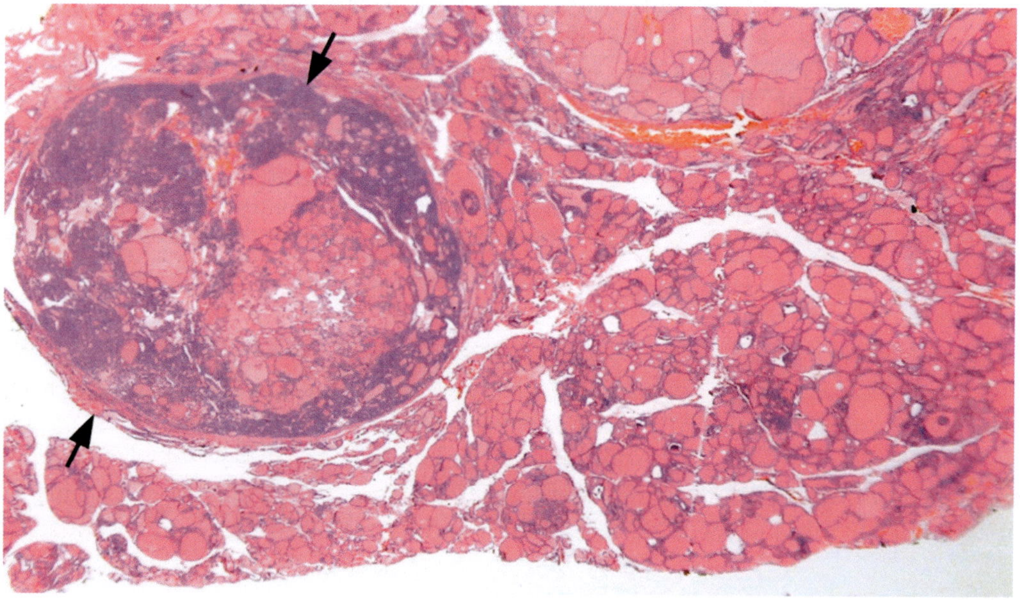

Fig 1.13 Adenomatoid nodule (arrows): with thin capsule in a background of nodular colloid goiter, the lesion comes in the differential diagnosis of follicular-patterned lesions

Macrofollicular variant of papillary carcinoma

This is a rare form of variant and is composed predominantly or exclusively of large follicles (not illustrated here). It is often confused with colloid or hyperplastic nodules or macrofollicular adenoma. The nuclear changes of PTC are always present. This variant is characterized by a low incidence of lymph node metastasis (40).

Tall cell variant of papillary carcinoma

Tall cell variant is defined as a tall-cell papillary carcinoma containing cells that are at least two times higher in height than width, and there must be 30% to 40% tall cells in the tumor (Fig.1.14 A, B). Necrosis, mitotic activity and extrathyroid extension are commonly seen and this variant shows more aggressive clinical behavior than in usual papillary carcinoma.(41). Most of th tall cell PTC show BRAF V600 mutations.

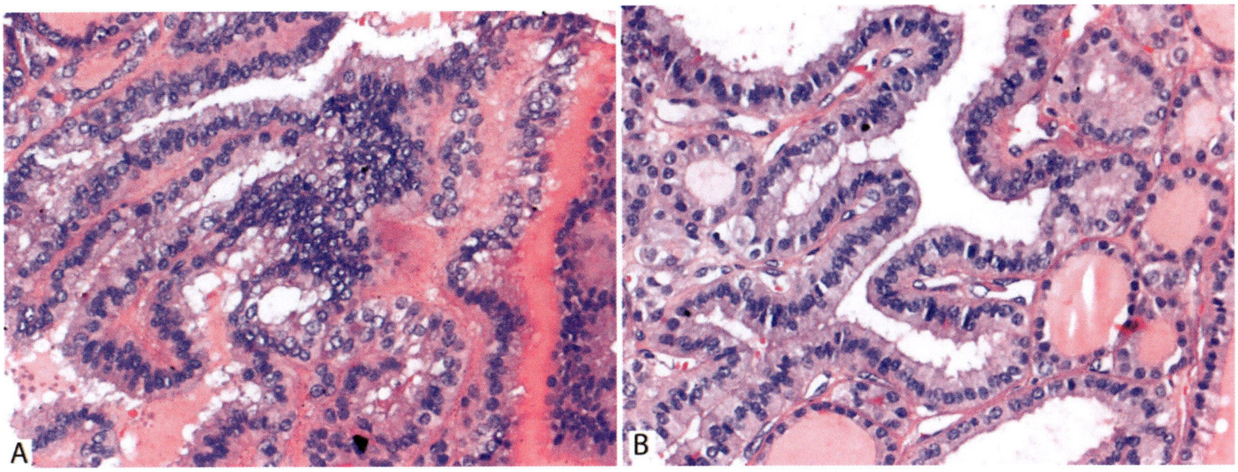

Fig 1.14 Tall cell variant of PTC: (A, B) tall cells (height of the cells twice the width of the cells) with papillary growth pattern

Diffuse Sclerosing Variant of PTC (DSVPTC)

The diffuse sclerosing variant of papillary thyroid carcinoma (DSVPTC) is an uncommon tumor making up about 2% of all papillary thyroid carcinomas. This variant mostly affects children and young adults and M:F ratio is 1.7:1.

Gross

The tumor shows diffuse replacement of the parenchyma by firm to hard white gritty tissue with variable extrathyroid extension.

Microscopic

Histologically, almost all cases demonstrate a papillary carcinoma (conventional, solid, or follicular pattern) diffusely involving the gland. Most cases show extrathyroid extension, lymphocytic thyroiditis, squamous metaplasia, increased fibrosis/sclerosis, many psammoma bodies and extensive lymphatic permeation (42). Dense hyalinized fibrosis often permeates widely within the tumor, dispersing small tumor islands. Both the papillary carcinoma and squamous metaplasia cells show immunoreactive with CK19, thyroglobulin, and TTF-1. Figure 1.15 (A, B, C, D) clearly show papillary nature of carcinoma and a very remarkable hyalinized fibrous stroma.

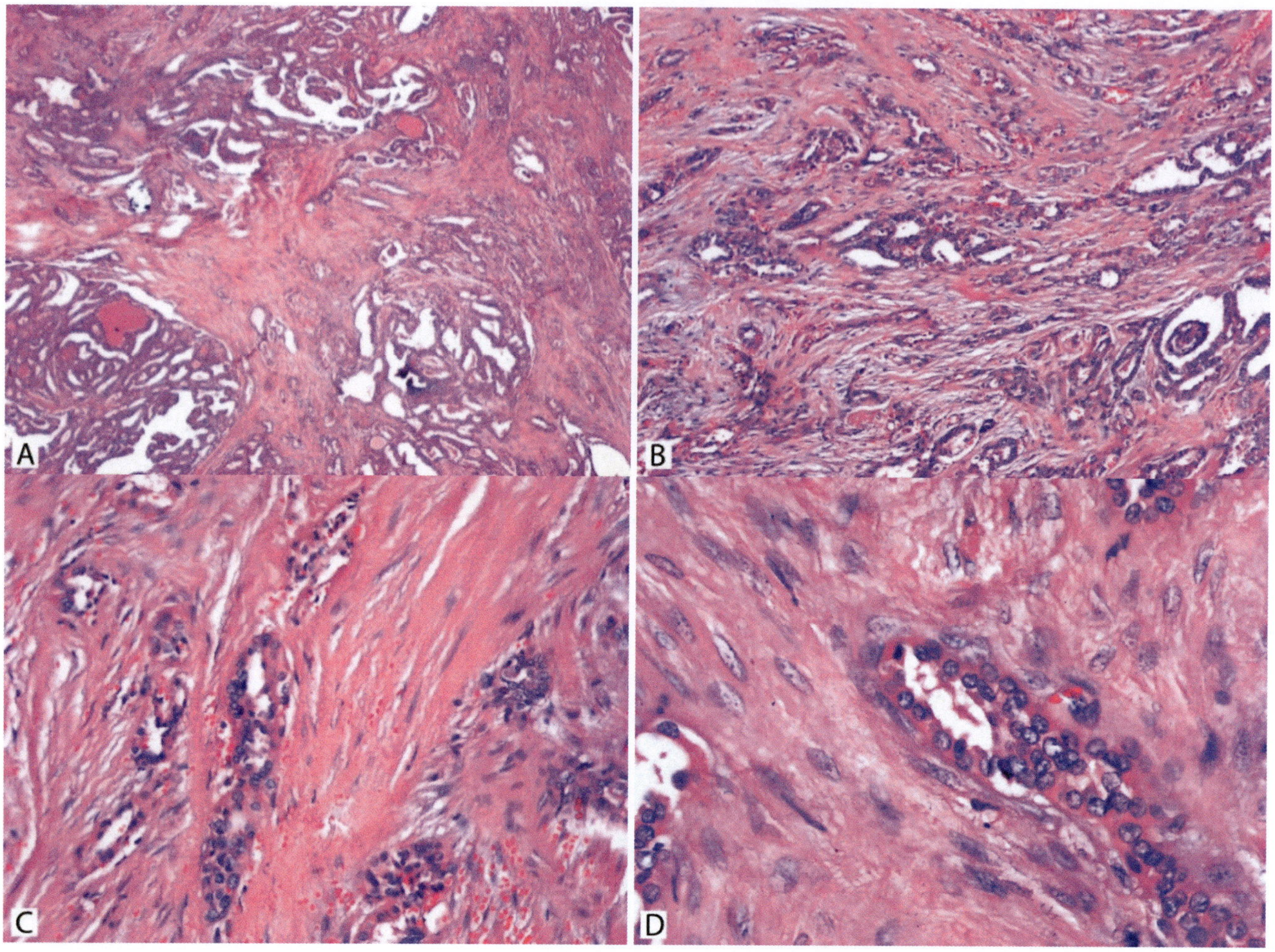

Fig 1.15 Diffuse sclerosing variant: (A) Scanner view shows solid foci of papillary carcinoma separated by thick hyalinized fibrous bands; (B, C, D) sclerotic fibrous tissue progressively separating single neoplastic units with some strangling effect

The tumor illustrated above is a papillary carcinoma with dense diffuse sclerosis. However, all the histological features illustrated in the literature on cases labelled as DSVPTC are not present in our case. Is our case to be labelled as the so called fibromatosis type (or nodular fasciitis type) of papillary thyroid carcinoma? Even for this entity published pictures are different in different articles on the subject. The authors feel that papillary thyroid carcinoma has many different morphological faces and some show a very conspicuous stromal reaction in the form of diffuse sclerosis or fibromatosis pattern. It is important to know that these variants of papillary carcinoma are more aggressive than conventional papillary thyroid carcinoma.

Prognosis

Many studies on the subject have shown that DSVPTC is an aggressive tumor with lymph node metastasis, extrathyroid extension and even pulmonary metastasis, seen more commonly than in conventional PTC (43). However, with aggressive multimodal therapy, the mortality is comparable with that of conventional PTC.

Variants with other patterns and composite patterns

Number of papillary carcinoma variants seems to be expanding and many are quite rare and often reported as single case reports. Variants with other patterns include oncocytic, clear cell, columnar cell, solid, cribriform, nodular fasciitis type etc. These cell types can be usually identified easily, even if seen for the first time.

Hyalinizing Trabecular Adenoma HTA

HTA, first identified by Carney et al (1987), is characterized by circumscription or encapsulation, trabecular-alveolar pattern of fusiform and polygonal tumor cells (Fig. 1.16 A, B, C), hyaline stroma, nuclei with prominent grooves, pseudoinclusions and psammoma bodies (44). The nuclear changes and psammoma bodies in HTA are similar to those encountered in papillary carcinoma. Some believe that hyalinising trabecular adenoma (HTA) is an encapsulated variant of papillary carcinoma because of some histological similarities: occasional occurrence of both tumors in the same gland, and similar pattern of expression of cytokeratins, including cytokeratin 19. The tumor may arise in a background of chronic lymphocytic thyroiditis, multinodular goiter, or may also occur in association with papillary thyroid carcinoma (45).

One study showed that HTA had minimal reactivity for cytokeratin 19 and no reactivity for high molecular weight keratin, whereas papillary carcinoma was strongly positive for these keratins (46). An occasional occurrence of cervical node metastasis of papillary carcinoma having HTA like pattern has been reported (47). There is a unique MIB1 (Ki-67) immunohistochemistry staining pattern noted in hyalinizing trabecular adenoma where there is a strong membranous and peripheral cytoplasmic reactivity, only identified with the Dako MIB1 antibody and not with those of other manufacturers. This pattern is helpful to confirm the diagnosis of hyalinizing trabecular adenoma.

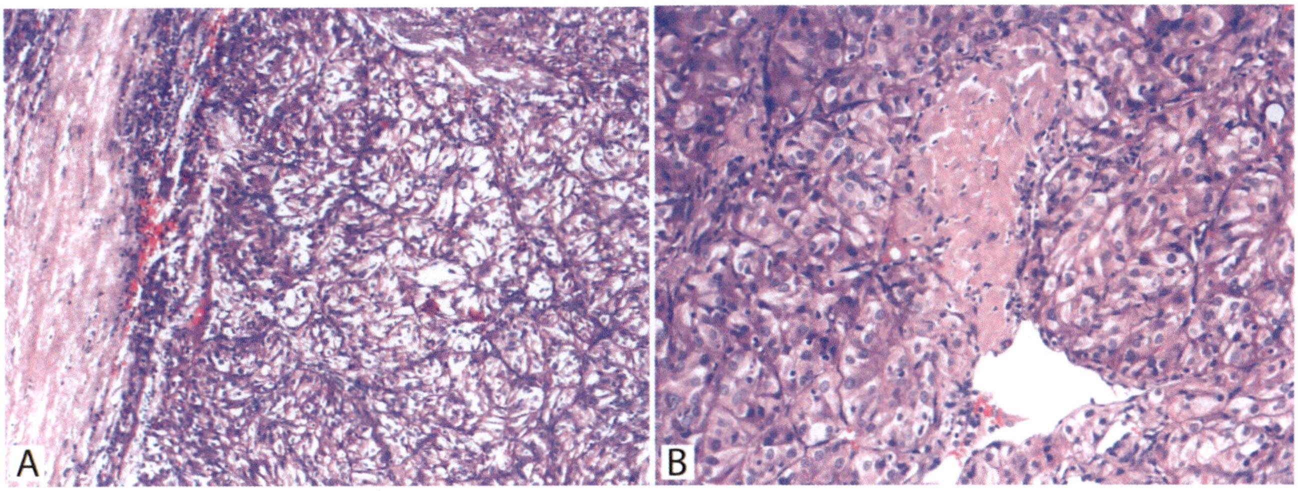

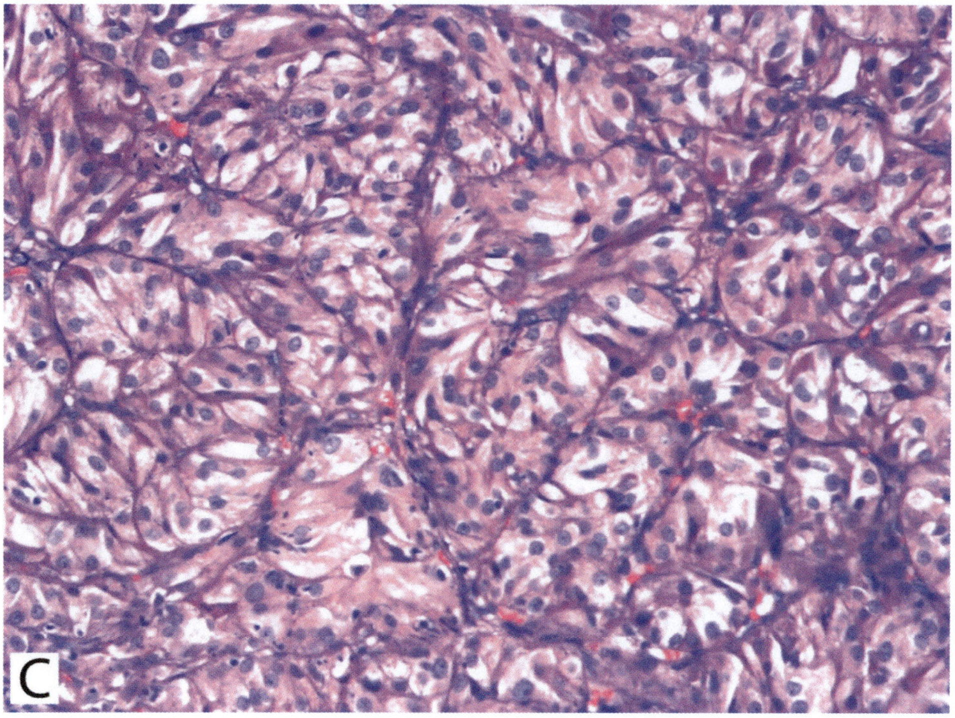

Fig 1.16 Hyalinizing trabecular tumor: (A) well encapsulated tumor; (B, C) typical alveolar and trabecular patterns; note hyalinized stromal band in (B)

Prognosis

The great majority of these tumors have behaved as benign neoplasms and should be treated as such. However, in view of controversy about its biological behavior, the term "hyalinized trabecular tumor" is preferred to "hyalinizing trabecular adenoma".

Hashmoto's Thyroiditis (HT) accompanied by papillary carcinoma or lymphoma (48)

Apart from relative rarity of malignant tumors arising in Hashimoto's thyroiditis, there are many fascinating attributes of this phenomenon, well brought about by an excellent review article on pathological analysis of 15,000 thyroidectomies carried out over a period of 124 years (1889-2012) at the Johns Hopkins hospital. Caturegli et al reported from this data, 867 cases of Hashimoto's thyroiditis, along with a total of 3591 malignant tumors of the thyroid over a period of 70 years (1942-2012) (48). The prevalence of Hashimoto's thyroiditis among a total 3394 cases of thyroid carcinoma was 251 cases (7.4%), of which 231 were papillary carcinomas and only 28 cases were of B cell lymphoma arisisng in HT. There were 867 cases.There are two very striking points from this work: (i) PTC occurs quite commonly in the milieu of chronic lymphocytic thyroiditis (231 in 867 cases of HT, 26.6%); (ii) Lymphoma rarely occurs in association with HT, only 28 cases (3.2%) of lymphoma were found among 867 cases of HT.

Papillary Thyroid Carcinoma in Hashimoto's Thyroiditis

In contemporary practice, pathology is rarely needed to establish a diagnosis of Hashimoto's thyroiditis and surgery is seldom used as a form of treatment. However, in this Johns Hopkins study, it is observed that incidence of surgical HT has significantly increased in the last two decades. The reason for surgical excision of thyroid is the frequent presentation of HT as a nodule rather than diffuse enlargement, which is diagnosed as suspicious of malignancy on FNAC.

It is debatable, whether the association represents co-occurrence of two relatively common conditions or indicates cause and effect relationship. In case of the latter, it is unclear whether cancer or autoimmunity comes first. Most recent studies suggest that papillary thyroid cancer follows a more benign course when accompanied by HT (48). Fig. 1.17 (A, B, C, D) shows a typical case of papillary carcinoma associated with Hashimoto's thyroiditis (HT)

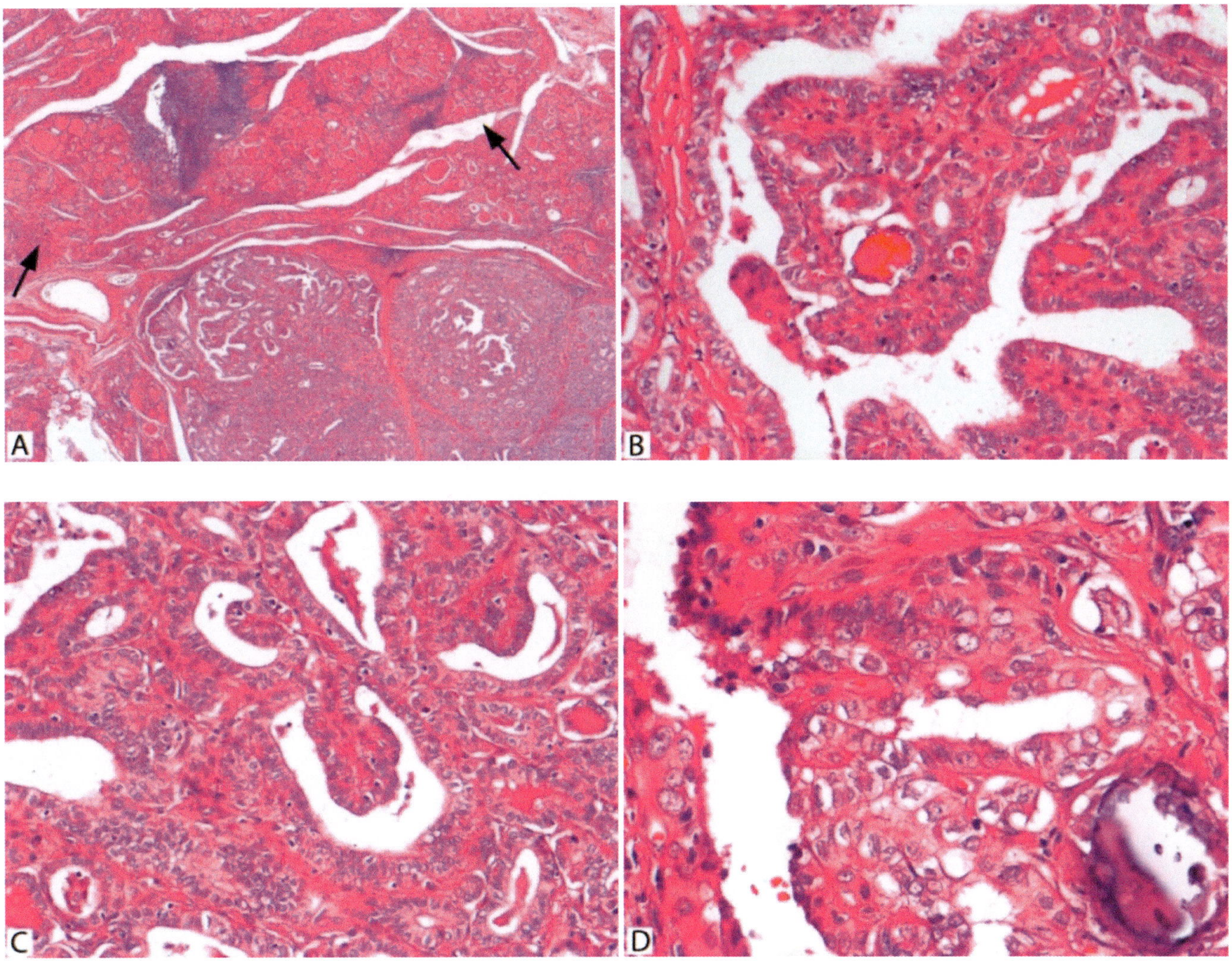

Fig 1.17 PTC in Hashimoto's: (A) Scanner view shows area of Hashimoto disease (arrows), note the presence of a papillary carcinoma growth in lower half); (B&C) close up of papillary patterns; (D) papillary carcinoma with calcified psammoma body.

Hashimoto's thyroiditis with primary malignant lymphoma (PTL)

In the case illustrated below masses of monomorphic lymphoid cells have replaced large areas of thyroiditis lesion and the tumor shows features of diffuse large B cell lymphoma (Fig 1.18 A-D) Malignant lymphoma may involve the thyroid as a part of systemic lymphoma or may arise as primary in the thyroid. Approximately 20% of patients dying of generalized malignant lymphoma will show thyroid involvement at autopsy (49). Various studies have shown that PTL typically occurs in the middle-aged to old-aged subjects with predilection for women, and arise in the setting of autoimmune thyroiditis (lymphocytic thyroiditis, Hashimoto's disease). The contribution of HT to papillary thyroid carcinoma remains controversial, but lymphoma of the thyroid is viewed as a consequence of long-standing autoimmune thyroiditis. The relative risk of developing lymphoma in patients with HT has been estimated to be 40-80 times greater than in the general population (50).

Derringer et al (51) reported a retrospective clinicopathologic study of 108 PTLs, classified using REAL and WHO classification schemes. There were 30 cases of marginal zone B cell lymphoma (MZBL), 36 cases of diffuse large B cell lymphoma (DLBCL) with MZBL, and 41 cases of DLBCL without MZBL. DLBCL and extranodal marginal zone B cell lymphoma of MALT type account for almost all cases of PTLs (52).

Cases with MZBL morphology and stage IE PTLs have excellent prognosis, whereas tumors with DLBCL component or stage greater than IE display poor prognosis.

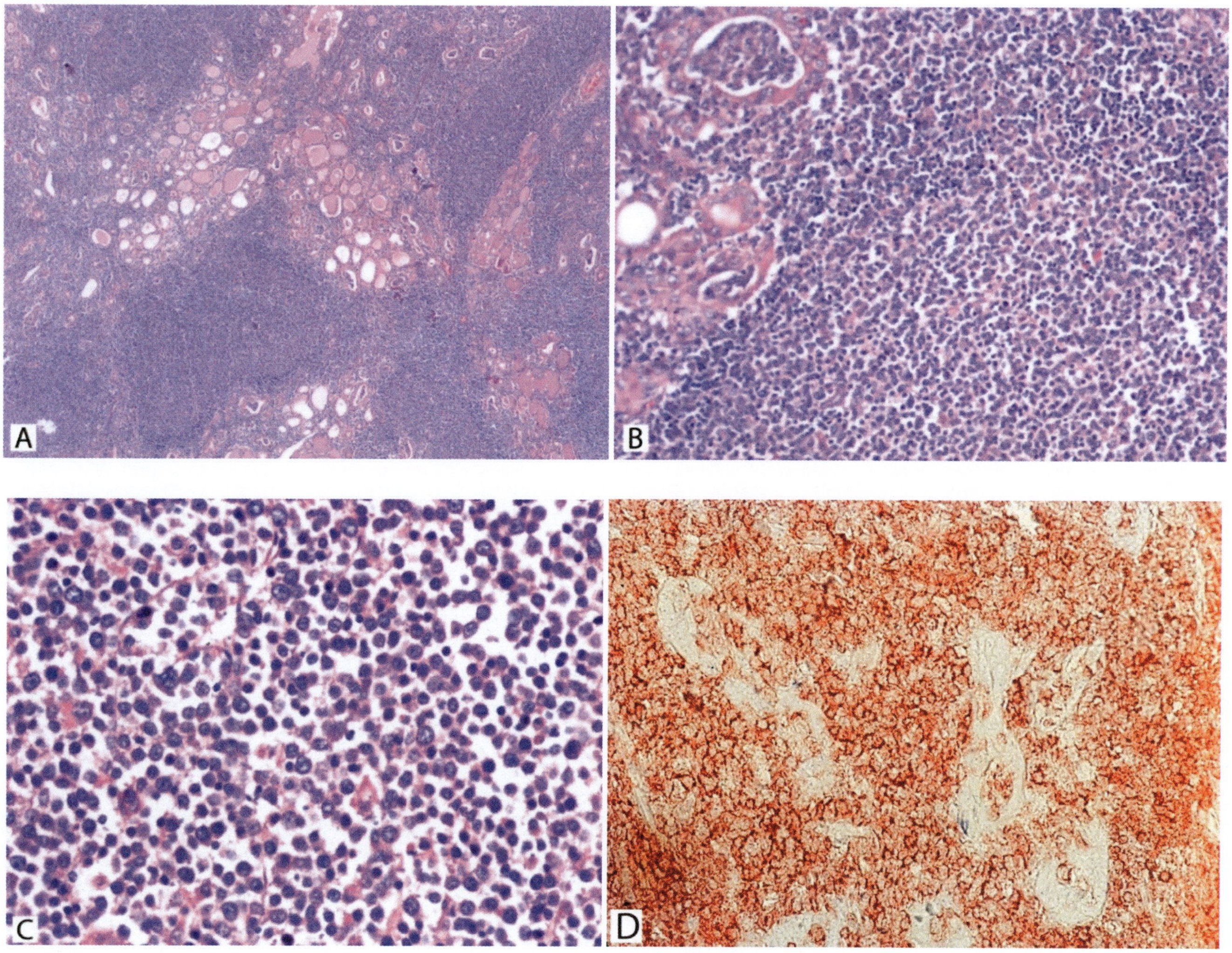

Fig 1.18 Lymphoma in Hashimoto's: (A) scanner view of Hashimoto's thyroiditis with marked lymphoid infiltrate and foci of atrophied thyroid acini containing Ashkenazy cells; (B) Ashkenazy cells along left border; (C) monomorphic large lymphoid cells; (D) neoplastic lymphoid cells strongly positive for CD20 immuno stain

Genetic testing for thyroid carcinoma

Primary screening of thyroid nodule is routinely accompanied by cytological evaluation of thyroid needle aspirated material. While, cytologic assessment is diagnostic in majority of patients, approximately, 15% to 20% biopies contain insufficient material of tissue for assessment and an additlional 15% to 20% have indeterminate cytological findings (54). Molecular diagnostics offers great promise for the evaluation of cytologically indeterminate thyroid nodules. Numerous molecular, genetic and immunohistochemical tests have been developed that may be performed on this aspirated thyroid material, which may greatly improve diagnostic yield (55). Identification of malignant tumors preoperatively would permit more extensive surgery, when indicated. Substantial developments have occurred in clinical translational research of thyroid cancer. Diagnostic molecular markers, such as, RET-PTC, Ras and BRAF V600E mutations, galectin 3; and a new gene expression classifier are outstanding examples that have improved diagnosis of thyroid nodules. For example, BRAF mutation is a prognostic genetic marker that has improved risk stratification and hence tailored management of patiets with thyroid cancer, including those with conventional low risks (54). Energetic molecular genetic testing has made inroads into the understanding of pathogenesis, differential diagnosis of follicular-patterened nodules and prognosis of differentiated thyroid cancer

Papillary Thyroid Carcinoma (PTC)

The V600E mutation of the BRAF gene is a common event in the papillary thyroid carcinoma and seems to play a key role in the development and progression of this disease. Results of a multicentaric study showed a strong association of BRAF with lymph metastasis, extrathyroid extension, advanced disease stages III and IV, and disese recurrence (55). The initial finding of the association of BRAF mutation with PTC recurrence is particularly relevant clinically, which has been confirmed by others (56). In view of the strong association of BRAF mutation with aggressiveness of PTC and the loss of radioiodine avidity of recurrent PTC (55), it seems prudent to surgically eradicate mutation positive PTC. Koperek et al (57) evaluated the expression of the mutated BRAF V600E protein in 144 cases of PTC using a novel mutation-specific antibody and found that 53% PTC showed diffuse cytoplasmic expression of the mutated BRAF protein. No statistical differernce in BRAF protein expression was seen between microcarcinomas and macrocarcinomas. American Thyroid Association recommended only lobectomy for microcarcinoma. But this new information suggests that total thyroidectomy may be carried out, if preoperative BRAF mutation is positive.

Follicular carcinoma & Follicular adenomas

Nikiforova and others (58) reported analyses of PAX8-PPARγ in a series of 118 thyroid tumors using a newly developed RT-PCR assay to detect this rearrangement in frozen and paraffin embedded tumor tissue. PAX8-PPARγ rearrangement was identified in follicular thyroid carcinomas but not in follicular adenomas or other thyroid tumors. Follicular carcinomas that were positive for PAX8-PPARγ rearrangement were often overtly invasive, whereas tumors negative for the rearrangement were typically minimally invasive.The presence of PAX8-PPARγ rearrangement in thyroid tumor cells detected by RT-PCR correlates with PPARγ immunohistochemical staining when only strong diffuse nuclear reactivity was scored positive.

Multi gene expression based testing:

A commercial multigene expression based classifier is available for clinical application using fine needle aspirations (FNA) cytology material. This 142 gene expression assay is used to classify indeterminate cytopathology interpretations including Follicular Lesion of Undetermined Significance (FLUS), Atypia of Undetermined Significance (AUS) and "suspicious for" Hürthle/Follicular Neoplasm into benign or malignant. Thus this provides definite preoperative diagnosis of a thyroid nodule and potentially reduces unnecessary surgery (59).

References

1) Bennedbaek FN, Hegedus L. Management of the solitary thyroid nodule: results of a North American Survey. J clin endocrinol metab 2000; 85:2493-2498

2) Gharib H, Goellner JR, Johnson DA. Fine-needle aspiration cytology of the thyroid: A 12-year experience with 11,000 biopsies. Clin Lab Med 1993; 13:669-709

3) LiVolsi VA, Albores-Saavedra J, Asa SL, et al Papillary carcinoma in DeLellis RA, Lloyd RA, Heitz PU, Charis E (Ed) Pathology and Genetics of Tumors of Endocrine Organs. WHO Classification of Tumors IARC Press Lyon 2004, P 57

4) Piana S, Frasoldati A, Felice E, et al. Encapsulated Well-differentiated Follicular-patterned Thyroid Carcinomas Do Not Play Significant Role in the Fatality Rates From Thyroid Carcinoma. Am J Surg Pathol 2010; 34:868-872

5) LiVolsi V. The demise of follicular carcinoma of the thyroid gland. Thyroid 1994; 4:233-236

6) Sobrinho Simose M, Asa SL, Kroll TG, et al Follicular carcinoma in DeLellis RA, Lloyd RA, Heitz PU, Charis E (Ed) Pathology and Genetics of Tumors of Endocrine Organs. WHO Classification of Tumors IARC Press Lyon 2004, P 68

7) Avanzo A, Treseler P, Iturate PHG, et al Follicular Thyroid Carcinoma: Histology and Prognosis. Cancer 2004; 100:1123-1129

8) Baloch ZW, LiVolsi VA. Follicular-patterned lesions of the thyroid. Am J Clin Pathol 2002; 117:143

9) Lin X, Zhu B, Liu Y, Silverman JF. Follicular thyroid carcinoma invades venous rather lymphatic vessels. Diagnostic Pathology 2010; 5:8-12

10) Baloch ZW, LiVolsi VA. Our approach to follicular-patterned lesions of the thyroid. J Clin Pathol 2007; 60:244-250

11) Sobrinho Simose M, Asa SL, Kroll TG, et al Follicular carcinoma in DeLellis RA, Lloyd RA, Heitz PU, Charis E (Ed) Pathology and Genetics of Tumors of Endocrine Organs. WHO Classification of Tumors IARC Press Lyon 2004, P 72

12) Johnson TL, Lloyd RV, Burney RE, et al. Hurthle Cell Thyroid Tumors: An Immunohistochemical study Cancer 1987; 59:107-112

13) Carcangiu ML, Bianchi S, Savino D, et al. Follicular Hurthle Cell Tumors of the Thyroid Gland. Cancer 1991; 68:1944-1953

14) Evans HL, Vassilopoulou R. Follicular and Hurthle Cell Carcinomas of the Thyroid: A Comparative Study. Am J Surg Pathol 1998; 22:1512-1520

15) Sakamoto A, Kasai N, Sugano H. Poorly differentiated carcinoma of the thyroid: A clinicopathologic entity for a high-risk group of papillary and follicular carcinoma

16) Carcangiu ML, Zampi G, Rosai J. Poorly differentiated ("insular") thyroid carcinoma. Am J Surg Pathol 1984; 8:655-668

17) Volante M, Collini P, Nikiforov YE, etc. Poorly differentiated thyroid carcinoma: The Turin proposal for the use of uninform diagnostic criteria and an algorithmic diagnostic approach. Am J Surg Pathol 2007; 31:1256-1264

18) Nishida T, Katayama, S, Tsujimoto, M, et al. Clinicopathologic Significance of Poorly Differentiated Thyroid Carcinoma Am J Surg Pathol 1999; 23:205-211

19) Dettmer M, Schmitt A, Steinert H, et al. Poorly differentiated Tbyroid Carcinomas: How much Poorly Differentiated is Needed? Am J Surg Pathol 2011; 35:1866-1872

20) Pilloti S, Collini P, Del Bp R, et al. A novel panel of antibodies that segregates immunohistochemically poorly differentiated carcinoma from undifferentiated carcinoma of the thyroid gland. Am J Surg Pathol 1994; 18:1054-1064

21) Carcangiu ML, SteeperT, Zampi G, et al. Anaplastic thyroid carcinoma: A study of 70 cases. Am J Clin Pathol 1985; 83:135

22) Agraval S, Rao RS, Parikh DM, et al. Histological trends in thyroid cancer1969-1993: A clinicopathologic analysis of relative proportion of anaplastic of the thyroid. J Surg Oncol 1996; 63:251-255

23) Demeter JG, De Jong SA, Lawrence AM, et al. Anaplastic thyroid carcinoma: risk factors and outcome Surgery 1991; 110:956-961

24) Hunt JL, Tometsko M, LiVolsi VA, et al. Molecular evidence of anaplastic transformation in co-existing well differentiated and anaplastic carcinomas of the thyroid Am J Surg Pathol 2003; 27:1559-1564

25) Venkaesh YSS, Ordonez AG, Schultz PN, et al Anaplastic carcinoma of the thyroid: A clinicopathologic study of 121 cases. Cancer 1990; 66:321-330

26) Patel KN, Shaha AR. Poorly Differentiated and Anaplastic Thyroid Cancer. Cancer Control 2006; 13:119-128

27) Wan SK, Chan JK, Tang SK. Paucellular variant of anaplastic thyroid carcinoma" A mimic of Riedel's thyroiditis Am j Clin Pathol 1995; 105:388-393

28) Rosai J, Zampi G, Carcangiu ML. Papillary carcinoma of the thyroid: A discussion of its several morphologic expressions, with particular emphasis on the follicular variant. Am J Surg Pathol 1983; 7:809-817

29) Carcangiu ML, Zampi G, Pupi A, et al. Papillary Carcinoma of the Thyroid: A clinicopathologic study of 241 cases treated at the University of Florence, Italy. Cancer 1985; 55:805-828

30) LiVolsi VA. Papillary neoplasms of the thyroid: Pathologic and prognostic features Am J clin Pathol 1992; 97:426-434

31) Mazafferri EL Young RL. Papillary thyroid carcinoma: a 10 year follow-up report of the impact of therapy in 576 patients. Am J Med 1981; 70:511-518

32) Fink A, Tomlinson G, Freeman JL, et al. Occult micropapillary carcinoma associated with benign follicular thyroid disease and unrelated thyroid neoplasms. Mod Pathol 1996; 9: 816-820

33) Hazard JB. Small papillary carcinoma of the thyroid: A study with special reference to so-called nonencapsulated sclerosing tumor. Lab Invest 1960; 9:86-97.

34. Woolner LB, Lemmon ML, Beahrs OH, et al. Occult papillary carcinoma of the thyroid gland: A study of 140 cases observed over a 30-year period. J Clin Endocrinol 1960; 2089-105.

35) Strate SM, Lee EL, Chik JH. Occult Papillary Carcinoma of the Thyroid With Distant Metastases. Cancer 1984; 54:1093-1100, 36) Min HS, Choe G, Kim SW, et al. S100A4 expression is associated with lymph node metastasis in papillary microcarcinoma of the thyroid. Mod Pathol 2008; 21:748-755

37) Liu J, Singh B, Tallini G, et al Follicular variant of papillary carcinoma: A clinicopathologic study of a problematic entity. Cancer 2006; 107:1255-1264

38 Chen KTK, Rosai J. Follicular variant of thyroid carcinoma: A clinicopathologic study of six cases. Am J Surg Pathol 1977; 1: 123-129

39) Kakudo K, Bai Y, Liu Z, et al. Encapsulated papillary thyroid carcinoma, a follicular variant: A misnomer. Pathology International 2012; 62:155-160

40) Albores-Saavedra J, Gould E, Vardaman C, et al. The macrofollicular variant of papillary thyroid carcinoma: a study of 17 cases Hum Pathol 1991; 221195-1205

41) Ostrowsky ML, Merino MJ. Tall cell variant of thyroid papillary carcinoma: a reassessment and immunohistochemical study with comparison to the usual type of papillary carcinoma. Am J Surg Pathol 1996; 20:864-974

42) Thompson LDR, Wieneke JA, Heffess CS. Diffuse sclerosing variant of papillary thyroid carcinoma: a clinicopathologic and immunophenotypic analysis of 22 cases. Endocr Pathol 2005; 16:331-348

42a) Heffess CS, Thompson LD. Minimally invasive follicular thyroid carcinoma. Endocr Pathol. 2001 Winter;12(4):417-22

43) Falvo L, Giacomelli L, D'Andrea V, et al. Prognostic importance of sclerosing variant in papillary thyroid carcinoma. The American Surgeon 2006; 72:438-444

44) Carney JA, Rayan J, Goellner JR. Hyalinizing trabecular adenoma of the thyroid gland. Am J Surg Path 1987; 11:583-591

45) Nose V, Volante M, Papotti M. Hyalinizing trabecular tumor of the thyroid: An update. Endocr Pathol 2008; 19:1-8

46) Hirokawa M, Carney JA, Ohtsuki Y. Hyalinising trabecular adenoma and papillary carcinoma of the thyroid express different cytokeratin patterns. Am J Surg Pathol 2000; 24:877-881

47) Li M, Rosai J, Carcangiu ML. Hyalinizing trabecular adenoma of the thyroid gland: A distinct tumor type or a pattern of growth? Modern Pathology 1995; 8:54A

48) Caturegli P, De Remigis A, Chuang K, et al 1). Hashimoto's Thyroiditis: Celebrating the Centennial Through the Lens of the Johns Hopkins Hospital Surgical Pathology Records. Thyroid 2012; 23:142-150

49) Binesh F, Akhavan A, Navabii H. Extranodal marginal zone B cell lymphoma of malt type with extensive plasma cell differentiation in a man with Hashimoto's thyroiditis. BMJ Case Reports 2011; doi 10.1136/bcr.052011.4277

50) Holm LE, Blomgren H, Lowhagan T. Cancer risks in patients with chronic lymphocytic thyroiditis. N Engl J Med 1985; 312:601-604

51) Derringer GA, Thompson LDR, Frommelt RA, et al. Malignant lymphoma of the thyroid gland: A clinicopathologic study of 108 cases. Am J Surg Pathol 2000; 24:623-639

52) Aozasa K, Inoue A, Tajima K et al. Malignant lymphomas of the thyroid gland: Analysis of 79 patients with emphasis on histologic prognostic factors. Cancer 1986; 58:100-104

(53) Kim N, Lavertu P. Evaluation of a thyroid nodule. Otolaryngol Clin North Am. 2003; 36:17–33

(54) Xing M, Haugen BR, Schlumberger M. Progress in molecular-based management of differentiated thyroid cancer. Lancet 2013; 381:1058-1069

(55) Xing M, Westra WH, Tufano RP, et al.BRAF mutation predicts a poorer clinical prognosis for papillary thyroid cancer J Clin EndocrinolMetab 2005; 90:6373-6379

(56) Elisei R, Viola D, Torregrossa L, et al. BRAF mutation is an independent, poor prognostic factor for the outcome of patients with low-risk intrathyroid PTC: single-institution results from a large cohort study. J Clin Endocrinol Metab 2012; 97: 4390-4398

(57) Koperek O, Kornouth C, Capper D, et al. Immunohistochemical detection of the BRAF V600E-mutated protein in papillary thyroid carcinoma. Am J Surg Pathol 2012; 36:844-850

(58) Nikiforova MN, Biddinger PW, Caudill CM, et al PAX8-PPAy rearrangement in thyroid tumors: RT-PCR and immunohistochemical analyses Am J Surg Pathol 2002; 26:1016-1023

(59) Alexander EK, et al. Preoperative Diagnosis of Benign Thyroid Nodules with Indeterminate Cytology. N Engl J Med. 2012;367:705-715.

Chapter 2 Parathyroid Carcinoma (PC)

Table 2.1 Lesions of Parathyroid glands (n = 199) Author's series (1970-2014)	
Adenoma	167 (83.9%)
Chief cell hyperplasia	21(10.5%)
Clear cell hyperplasia	2(1%)
Carcinoma	7 (3.5%)
Simple cysts	2 (1%)

Introduction

Parathyroid carcinoma is an exceedingly rare clinical entity, accounting for only 0.5% to 2 % cases of patients with primary hyperparathyroidism. It is the least common endocrine malignancy and accounted for 0.005% of 286 cases of PC reported to the US National Cancer Database (NCDB) (1). PC occurs equally in males and females with a mean age of 45 years. More than 90% of patients present with symptoms of hyperparathyroidism. The relative incidence of proliferative processes giving rise to primary hyperparathyroidism: carcinoma in 0.5 to 2%, adenomas in 85% and diffuse hyperplasia in 10% (2).

Approximately 290 cases of parathyroid carcinoma were reported in the English literature between 1930 and 1992. Since 1992, more than 100 additional cases have been reported (3)

Etiology

Many cases of PC have been reported in patients with a history of neck irradiation for unrelated disease (3).

Few cases of PC have been reported to have arisen from parathyroid adenoma or hyperplasia of parathyroid (4).

PC has been described in patients with end stage renal disease and those on long term hemodialysis (5). Overactivity of the parathyroid gland with both hyperplasia and adenoma is present even in early stages of chronic renal failure. PC apparently arises from initially benign lesions of parathyroid glands

PC has been shown to be associated with multiple endocrine neoplasia type 1, albeit rarely. Hyperparathyroidism is the most common manifestation in patients with MEN 1, reaching a prevalence of 100% by age of 40 years; it is usually due to chief cell hyperplasia or adenoma (6).

Clinical findings

The clinical features of parathyroid carcinoma are due primarily to the effects of excessive secretion of parathormone by the functioning tumor rather than to infiltration of tissues in the neck. The challenge to the clinician lies in differentiation of hyperparathyroidism due to parathyroid carcinoma and that due to much more common adenoma/hyperplasia lesion. All too often the diagnosis of PC is made in retrospect when hypercalcemia recurs due to local spread of tumor or distant metastasis. Schantz and Castleman (1973) reported in a series of 70 cases, signs and symptoms with following frequency: bone disease 62%, palpable neck mass 31%, urolithiasis 30%, and parenchymal renal disease 21% (7). On the other hand, primary hyperparathyroidism due to adenoma/hyperplasia usually presents with mild hypercalcemia, typically within 1 mg/dL above the upper limit of normal.

The high levels (thousands of pg/ml) of parathormone in PC lead to a severe degree of hypercalcemia, which is invariably associated with typical signs and symptoms of hypercalcemia. The most frequent complaints are fatigue, weakness, weight loss, anorexia, nausea, vomiting, polyuria and polydipsia. Other presenting signs characteristic of severe hyperparathyroid state, include bone pain, fractures, renal colic, nephrolithiasis and renal insufficiency. In fact, simultaneous overt renal and bone involvement is distinctly unusual in hyperparathyroidism following adenoma or hyperplasia (1).

It cannot be too strongly reiterated that detailed knowledge of clinical findings in hyperparathyroidism is essential, since histological diagnosis of parathyroid carcinoma and adenoma is indeed difficult.

Gross

In contrast to soft tan white or reddish grey 1to 3 cm sized adenoma, carcinomas are firm grey white with occasional focus of necrosis. In addition, carcinomas are large tumors, that are often adherent to the surrounding structures. In fact, the presence of a grey white parathyroid mass with macroscopic evidence of fibrosis, particularly when associated with calcium >14 should prompt an en clock resection of tumor with ipsilateral thyroid lobe, soft tissues of neck and adjacent nodes. The option of radical surgical resection is thus, driven purely on gross findings.

Microscopic

(Fig 2.1 A-E & 2,2 A-D)

The principle histologic features that distinguish parathyroid carcinoma from adenoma are a trabecular pattern, thick fibrous bands, mitotic figures, and capsular and vascular invasion (7). Other histologic findings are tumor cell monotony, increased N/C ratio, spindling of tumor cells, prominent irregular macronuclei and focal necrosis. Examination of frozen sections and electron microscopic studies are of little value in distinguishing benign from malignant.

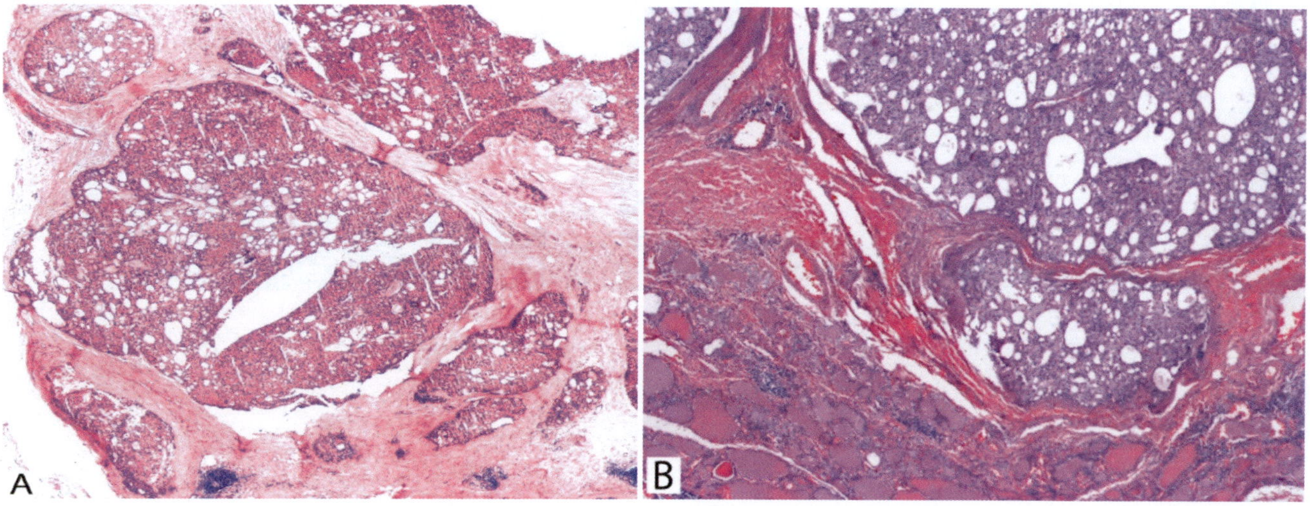

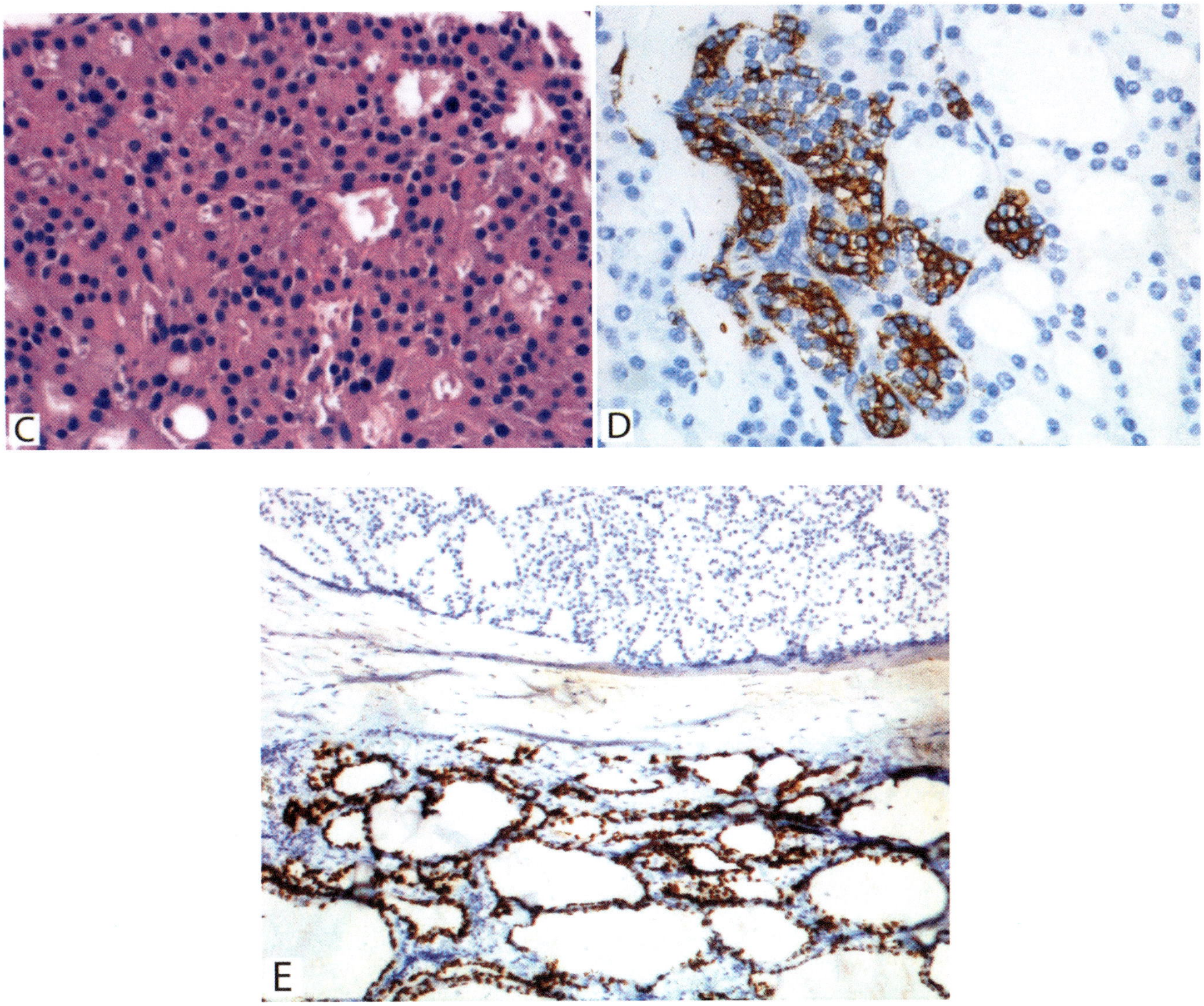

Fig 2.1 Parathyroid carcinoma: (A) scanner view shows PC with multifocal invasion in the surrounding neck soft tissues; (B) In this picture tumor island has invaded adjacent thyroid; (C) high power showing neoplastic chief cells with dense hyperchromatic but bland nuclei with no mitosis; (D) positive chromogranin staining of clusters of tumor cells; (E) TTF1 strongly positive in thyroid follicular cells but not in the parathyroid tumor above (Courtsy: Dr Jay Mehta, SRL Diagnostics, Mumbai, has kindly contributed this case of parathyroid carcinoma).

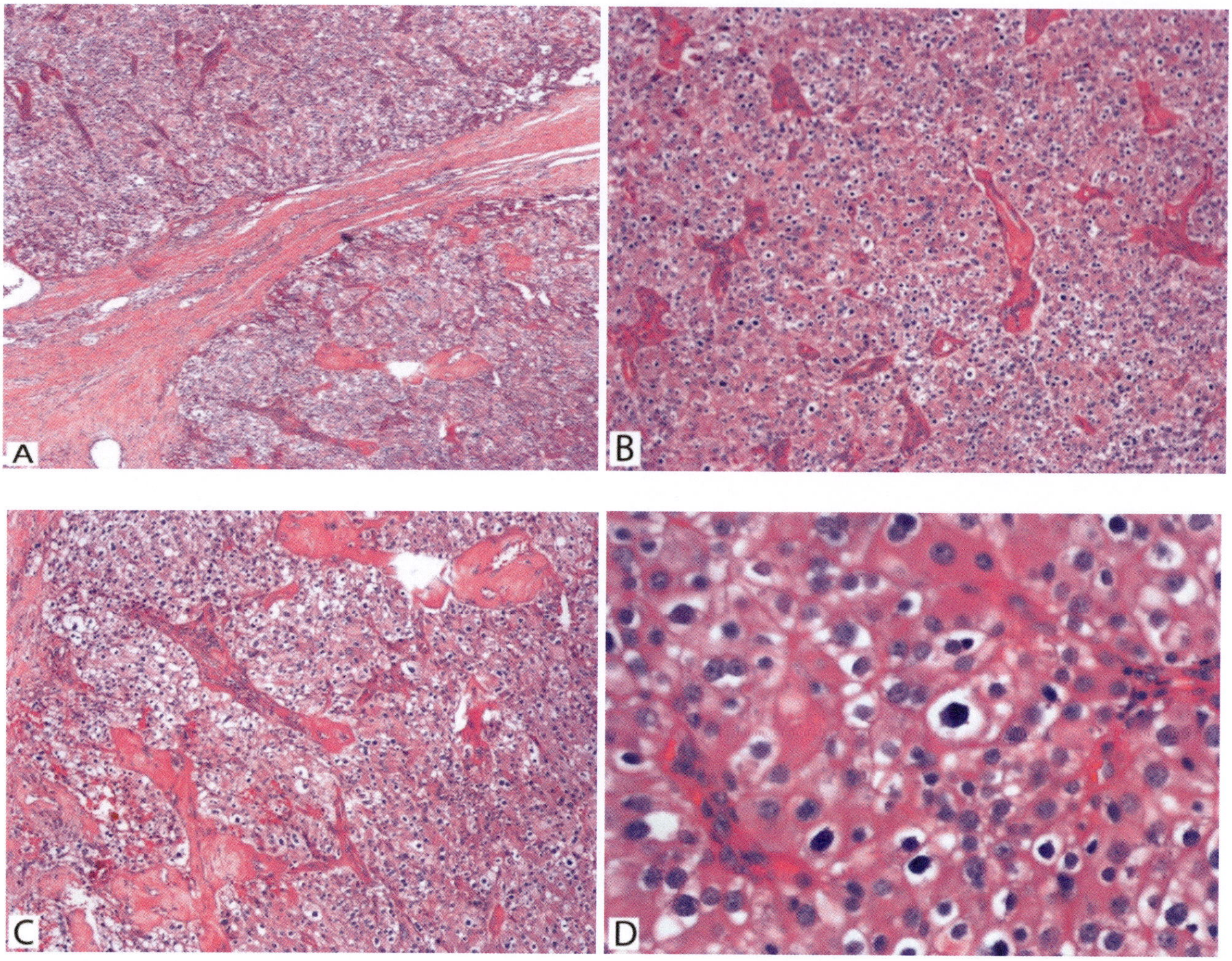

Fig 2.2 Another case of PC: (A) right lower third portion is the tumor and left upper third is extension to the exterior; (B,C) short fibrous septa around nests of tumor cells; (D) high power of chief cells with vacuolated or acidophilic cytoplasm and enlarged hyperchromatic and pleomorphic nuclei.

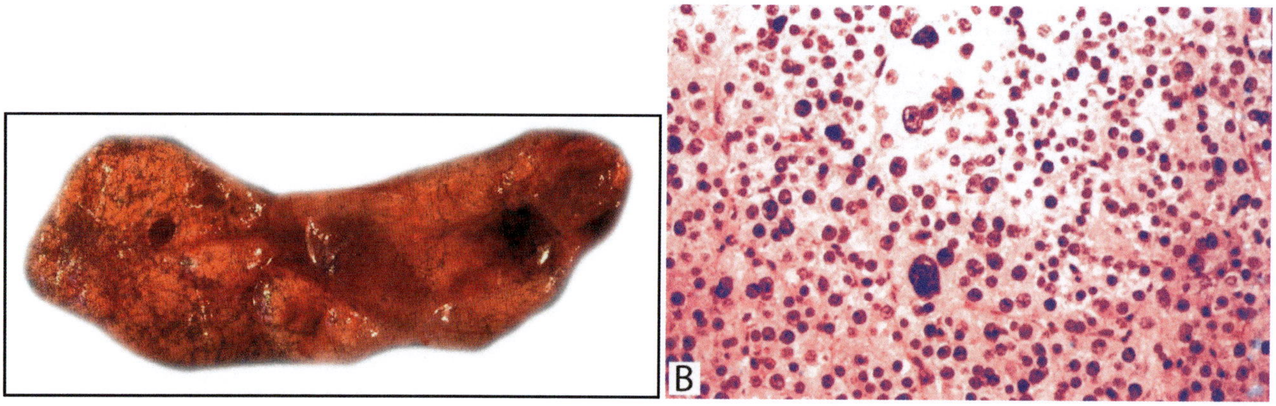

Fig 2.3 Parathyroid adenoma for comparison: (A) orange brown encapsulated adenoma; (B) high power picture with nuclear pleomorphism, no mitosis

Many microscopic features in favour of carcinoma are listed above but only invasion in surrounding tissues and vascular invasion are reliable criteria. All others parameters, including some nuclear pleomorphism, can also be seen in adenomas.

In an excellent clinical review of 122 cases of hyperthyroidism, Shane (3) has tabulated clinical, biochemical and pathological features of hyperthyroidism associated with parathyroid carcinomaVersus those associated with hyperplasia/adenoma. This information is extremely useful to distinguish parathyroid carcinoma from benign parathyroid lesions clinically and intraoperatively. An early recognition and prompt radical surgery will greatly improve "cure" or long term survival in parathyroid carcinoma. In PC with hyperparathyroidism, F: M ratio was 1:1, serum calcium >14 mg, parathormone markedly elevated, palpable mass in neck, renal involvement in 33% and skeletal involvement in 62% . Whereas, hyperparathyroidism due to hyperplasia/adenoma showed 3.5:1 F: M ratio, serum calcium >1 mg, almost no palpable neck mass, and minimal renal or skeletal involvement. Introperatively, PC presents thick adherent capsule and even infiltration in soft tissues of neck whereas adenoma (Fig 2.3 A,B) presents as a smooth encapsulated easily excised nodule

Prognosis

The prognosis of parathyroid carcinoma is quite variable. No one characteristic correlates predictably with outcome. Early recognition and complete resection at the time of initial surgery carry the best prognosis. The average time between surgery and the first recurrence is approximately 3 years, although intervals of up to 20 years have been reported. Once the tumor has recurred, complete cure is unlikely, although prolonged survival is still common with palliative surgery (3). Although complete, en block resection of all tumor represents the best opportunity for cure, a substantial proportion of patients fail to receive such treatment. The rarity of PC and late intraoperative recognition apparently prevent optimal treatment.

A National Cancer Data Base report showed that overall survival at 5 years and 10 years is 85.5% and 49% respectively. At 5-years of follow up and possibly beyond, neither tumor size nor lymph node size were found to be significant prognostic factors (1).

References

1) Hundahl SA, Fleming ID, Fremgen AM, et al. Two hundred eighty-six cases of parathyroid carcinoma treated in the US between 1985-1995: A National Cancer Data Base Report Cancer 1999; 86:538-544

2) Wilkins B, Lewis JS. Non-functional parathyroid carcinoma: A review of the literature and report of a case requiring extensive surgery Head & Neck Pathol 2009; 3:140-149

3) Shane E. Clinical review 122 Parathyroid Carcinoma. J Clin Endocrinol Metab 2001; 86:485-493

4) Kauffmann R, Juhlin C, Fohn LE, et al. Parathyroid carcinoma arising from four gland hyperplasia. Endocr Pract 2011; 17:1-9

5) Berland Y, Olmer M, Lebreuil G, et al Parathyroid carcinoma, adenoma and hyperplasia in a case of chronic renal insufficiency on dialysis Clin Nephrol 1982; 18:154-158

6) Kodroff KS, Lieber C, Thompson LDR. Parathyroid carcinoma occurring in multiple endocrine neoplasia type 1. Endocr Pract 1999; 5:347-349

7) Shantz A, Castleman B. Parathyroid Carcinoma: A study of 70 cases. Cancer 1973; 31:600-605

Chapter 3: Gastro-Entero-Pancreatic Endocrine Tumors

The Dispersed Neuroendocrine System

Introduction

Oberndorfer in 1907 described special tumors of the small intestines, which he called "Karzinoide Tumoren" (carcinoids) (1). Little did he realize that his discovery will lead to an uncharted territory, the 'dispersed neuroendocrine system'. The journey from carcinoid to neuroendocrine system has been fascinating, tortuous, long, and spanning a period of nearly 100 years after the seminal contribution of Oberndorfer. The nervous system comprises the conventional somatic and autonomic divisions and now includes the neuroendocrine system. The neuroendocrine cells occur in pituitary, adrenal medulla, thyroid (C cell), parathyroid, paraganglia, broncho-pulmonary and gastrointestinal endocrine cells, pancreatic islets, Merkel cell of skin and miscellaneous sites such as breast, cervix, prostate, larynx etc. And some of the unusual primary sites include kidney, paranasal sinuses, liver, gall bladder, middle ear, eye, orbit and mesentery. (1)

Origin of Neuroendocrine Cells

Feyrter (1938) suggested that the GI endocrine cells formed an integral part of a diffuse endocrine system, in which constituent cells are diffusely scattered in singles or small groups throughout the tissues of the body. He believed that the endocrine cells arose from the mucosa of the gut and is, therefore, derived from the endoderm (2). Pearse (1969) described the cytochemical characteristics of the cells of the dispersed neuroendocrine system (DNS) and coined the acronym 'APUD' (Amine Precursor Uptake Decarboxylase). He propounded that the cells, to be called neuroendocrine cells, arose from the neural crest and migrated to various sites in alimentary and respiratory systems, and conventional endocrine organs.(3)

The subject of embryological derivation of neuroendocrine cells of the gastrointestinal and respiratory system is controversial but now it is accepted that the endocrine cells of gastrointestinal tract and pancreas are derived from specialized cells in the embryonic GI system (endoderm), which can differentiate into endocrine and acinar cells. The neural crest origin of cells of the anterior pituitary, thyroidal C cells, chromaffin cells of adrenal medulla and certain cells of paragangliomas is well accepted. It is futile to ponder over the exact embryological origin of neuroendocrine cell. Instead, we should focus on the amalgamation of the neural and endocrine physiologic mechanisms which are integral to the neuroendocrine system (4).

Definition of Neuroendocrine cells

These are cells that receive neuronal input (transmitters released by nerve cells) and, as a consequence of this input, release message molecules (hormones) to the blood. In this way they bring about integration between nervous system and the endocrine system, a process known as neuroendocrine integration.

Identification of Neuroendocrine Cells

All neuroendocrine cells are readily identified by immunohistochemical staining for neuron-specific enolase (NSE), chromogranin and synaptophysin. In all suspected cases of neuroendocrine tumors, these stains are regularly employed and found to be consistently positive and reliable. Electron microscopy invariably shows dense core neurosecretory granules measuring from 150 to 400 nm in size in all neuroendocrine cells and their lesions.

Nomenclature

Neuroendocrine cells and their tumors are subdivided into hormonally functioning and non-functioning types. The hormone secreting neuroendocrine tumors are labeled according to the type of the hormone secreted or presenting clinical syndromes (for example insulinoma, see Table 3.1)

Enterochromaffin (EC) cells (Kulchitsky cells) are a type of enteroendocrine cells occurring in the epithelial lining of the digestive tract and the respiratory tract and contain about 90% of the body's store of serotonin (5-Hydroxy tryptamine). The cells are stimulated by gastrin molecule that is produced in the antrum of the stomach by G cells.

The other population of chromaffin cells found only in the stomach is called enterochromaffin-like cells (ECL). They look like EC cells but do not contain 5-HT. ECL cells respond to gastrin released by G-cells and release histamine which stimulates parietal cells to secrete gastric acid.

Anatomical Distribution and Functions of Cells of Neuroendocrine System

Hormones of gastro-entero-pancreatic endocrine system are all peptides and as of 1925 three peptides, namely secretin, gastrin and cholecystokinin (CCK) were described. The list of peptides has grown exponentially to over 30 peptides in the last 5 decades. The anatomical location and functions of various cells are tabulated below.

Table 3.1: Established Peptide Hormones

	Distribution	Functions
Cholecystokinin diminishing towards ileum	Numerous in duodenum, moderate in jejunum	stimulates contraction of gall bladder and pancreatic secretions
Secretin	Concentration highest in duodenum followed by Jejunum	stimulates pancreatic bicarbonate secretion and counteracts duodenal acidification
Gastric Inhibitory Peptide [GIP]	Duodenum and jejunum	inhibits secretion of gastric acid enhances insulin secretions
Enkephalin	Found through out the gut Particularly in antrum & upper duodenum	increases muscle tone & gastric emptying, controls pain
Motilin	Widely distributed in GI tract from esophagus To anus, also gall bladder and biliary tract	controls activity of gastrointestinal musculature
Substance P	Through out GI tract with highest in small bowel, Also in central & peripheral nervous systems	stimulates intestinal peristalsis; modulates esophageal sphincter & gall bladder contraction

Table 3.2: Peptide Hormones Associated with Syndromes

	Distribution	Functions
Gastrin [G cells]	Largest population found in gastric antrum Duodenum major source of extra-antral Gastrin	Major action: stimulation of HCL secretions from parietal cells; also stimulates pepsin and intrinsic factor
Glucagon [A cells]	Exclusively in alpha cells of islets Of Langerhans Glucagon imunoreactivity found in certain Intestinal and neural cells but do not secrete Glucagon	Glycogenolysis and gluconeogenesis in liver
Insulin [B cells]	Exclusively secreted by beta cells of islets Of Langerhans	Increases glucose intake & utilization, increases lipogenesis, general anabolic Effect
Pancreatic Polypeptides [PP]	Cells in periphery of islets of head of pancreas & dispersed in exocrine Pancreas	Suppression of exocrine pancreatic secretions & gall bladder contractions
Somatostatin {D Cell]	Found throughout the central nervous, gastrointestinal and genitourinary systems Also found in thyroid, adrenal medulla thymus, spleen & salivary glands, highest. Concentration in duodenum & pancreas, also In myenteric plexuses and mucosa of GI tract	Widespread inhibitory actions on GI tract pituitary and pancreatic peptides; inhibits release of gastrin, secretin, CCK, GIP Motilin, VIP, insulin, glucagon, pancreatic PP, growth hormone & TSH
Vasoactive Intestinal Peptide [VIP]	Concentrated mainly in GI tract with large amounts in the nerves of intestinal wall; also Found in brain and genitourinary tract	Most important function is vasodilatation, smooth muscle contraction and secretions of intestinal and genitourinary tracts

Neuroendocrine tumors of gastrointestinal tract and pancreas

General Considerations (Tables 3.3, 3.4)

The term carcinoid is well entrenched in the medical literature and is synonymous with the term neuroendocrine tumor. The term APUDOMA, which also means carcinoid/neuroendocrine tumor, is now abandoned. WHO 2000 on neuroendocrine classification retained the term carcinoid but, 2003 WHO classification has replaced this term with endocrine tumor/endocrine carcinoma.

The tumors arising from neuroendocrine cells are all identical morphologically, regardless of the anatomical site and whether functional or nonfunctional. The functioning tumor is identified on the basis of clinical presentation and determination of hormone level in blood by RIA.

Table 3.3: Classification of Gastro-entero-pancreatic Endocrine Tumors

Stomach	Cell of origin	Main hormone produced
Carcinoid tumor type I	ECL	Histamine
Carcinoid tumor type II	ECL	Histamine
Carcinoid tumor type III	ECL	Histamine
Gastrinoma	G	Gastrin
Duodenum		
Gastrinoma	G	Gastrin
Somatostatinoma	D	Somatostatin
Gangliocytic paraganglioma	?	Somatostatin, PP
Carcinoid tumor	EC	Serotonin
Small intestine & cecum		
Carcinoid tumor	EC	Serotonin
Rectum & sigmoid colon		
Carcinoid tumor	EC	Serotonin
Pancreas		
Insulinoma	B cell	Insulin
Gastrinoma	G cell	Gastrin
Glucagonoma	A cell	Glucagon
VIPoma	not known	Vasoactive intestinal peptide
Somatostatinoma	D cell	Somatostatin, ACTH, Calcitonin etc

(Kloppel G, Perren A, Heitz PU: The Gastroenteropancreatic Neuroendocrine Cell System and Its Tumors: The WHO classification. Ann. N. Y. Acad. Sci 2004; 1014:13-27) (5)

Table 3.4: Grading of Gastro-entero-pancreatic endocrine tumors	
(A) Well differentiated endocrine tumor	
Grade I (Benign behavior)	Non-functioning, histologically bland, <1 cm Mucosa-submucosa, non-angioinvasive
Grade II (malignancy uncertain)	Non-functioning, histologically bland,1-2 cm Mucosa-submucosa, sometimes angioinvasive
(B) Well differentiated endocrine carcinoma	
Grade III (low grade malignant)	Sometimes functional, bland, >2 cm, extension beyond submucosa, with or without angioinvasion
(C) Poorly differentiated endocrine carcinoma	
Grade IV (high grade malignant)	Cytologically poorly differentiated, some functioning others not functioning, poor prognosis

(Kloppel G, Perren A, Heitz PU: The Gastroenteropancreatic Neuroendocrine Cell System and Its Tumors: The WHO classification. Ann. N. Y. Acad. Sci 2004; 1014:13-27) (5)

Prevalence of Neuroendocrine tumors of digestive system

Modlin et al presented a 5-decade analysis of 13,715 carcinoid tumors, which represents the largest epidemiology series addressing carcinoid tumors from various sites in the body (Table 3.5)(6).

Table 3.5 Prevalence of carcinoid tumors	
Site	**No of Cases**
Small intestine	3938 (41.8%)
Rectum	2581 (27.4%)
Appendix	1679 (17.8%)

(Adapted from Modlin IM, Lye KD, Kidd M: A 5-decade Analysis of 13,715 Carcinoid Tumors. Cancer 2003; 97: 934-959 (6)

Neuroendocrine Tumors (NET) of Stomach

Definition

The majority of endocrine tumors of the stomach are well differentiated, non-functioning enterochromaffin-like (ECL) cell carcinoids arising from oxyntic mucosa of the gastric body and fundus.

Clinical Findings

Neuroendocrine tumors of the stomach arise from enterochromaffin like cells (ECL), and NETs from all other sites in GI tract arise from enterochromaffin cells (EC). ECL cells secrete histamine, while EC cells secrete serotonin. EC cell carcinoid is extremely rare in stomach and hence gastric carcinoid tumors do not give rise to Carcinoid Syndrome. On the basis of pathophysiology, three types of ECL cell gastric carcinoids are identified (7, 8)

Type 1) Autoimmune chronic atrophic gastric or treatment with proton pump inhibitors, which destroy parietal cells giving rise to achlorhydria and hypergastrinemia (Diagram 1)

Type 2) Associated with multiple endocrine neoplasia (MEN 1) and Zollinger-Ellison syndrome with associated gastrinoma producing hypergastrinemia (Diagram 1)

Type 3) Occurring sporadically (spontaneous) and not associated with hypergastrinemia.

Microscopic

It is necessary to know the various cell types normally occurring in gastric glands of fundus and body of stomach (Table 3.6) in order to understand the pathogenesis of ECL cell carcinoid and its surrounding milieu.

Table 3.6: Cells of Gastric Glands and Secretory products	
Chief cell	Pepsinogen
Parietal cell	Acid, Intrinsic factor
Endocrine Cells	
G cells (mainly antral)	Gastrin
D cells (sparse & central)	Somatostatin
ECL cell	Histamine (Fundus & body)

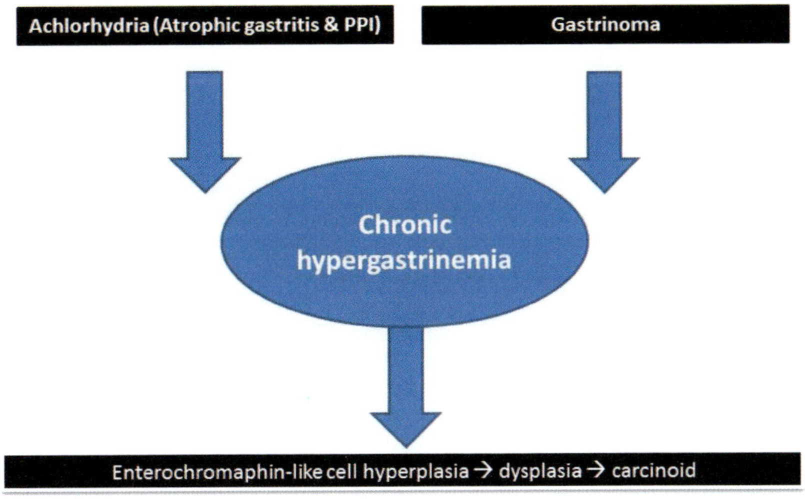

Diagram 1: modified and adopted from, Bordi C, D'Adda T, Azzoni C, Ferraro G: Pathogenesis of ECL tumors in humans. Yale J Biol Med. 2003; 71: 273-284 (9)

Type 1 gastric carcinoids

In autoimmune gastritis, circulating auto antibodies cause selective destruction of acid secreting parietal cells, which lead to a state of hypergastrinemia. This also occurs in proton pump inhibitor drugs used in cases for therapeutic reduction of gastric acid and in cases of H pylori induced severe chronic gastritis. Hypergastrinemia will give rise to small nodules of ECL cell hyperplasia, which may lead to dysplasia and eventually carcinoid tumor. Type 1 carcinoids appear as tan nodules or polyps within the mucosa, majority <1 cm, and are multiple in 57% of cases (Figure. 3.1). Bulk of Type 1 gastric carcinoids behave in an entirely benign fashion, a few will invade the muscularis propria (Figure 1B, IC). (10, 11, 12, 13,14)

Type 2 gastric carcinoids (Zollinger Ellison Syndrome)

These arise from ECL cells in the body mucosa in a background of ECL cell hyperplasia secondary to a gastrin producing carcinoid in the duodenum or pancreas. About 20% of cases of ZES are associated with MEN 1 syndrome. The risk of development of Type 2 carcinoid is almost 100 times greater in MEN 1 associated ZES than in sporadic ZES. The mortality for Type 2 is largely dependent on the stage of associated gastrinoma but is about 10%

Type 3 gastric carcinoids of EC cells

They are rather uncommon in stomach and are often bulky tumors with local lymph node metastases at presentation. Transmural invasion and serosal involvement are commonly seen. This tumor is akin to small cell undifferentiated or "oat" cell bronchogenic carcinoma in its structure and behavior. The mortality rate for Type 3 carcinoid is in the range of 25%-30%

A particularly aggressive gastric neuroendocrine tumor has been described. These are heterogeneous with multidirectional differentiation - combined glandular and endocrine components. Transmural invasion, serosal infiltration and metastasis to regional lymph nodes are often seen at the time of presentation.(14, 15)

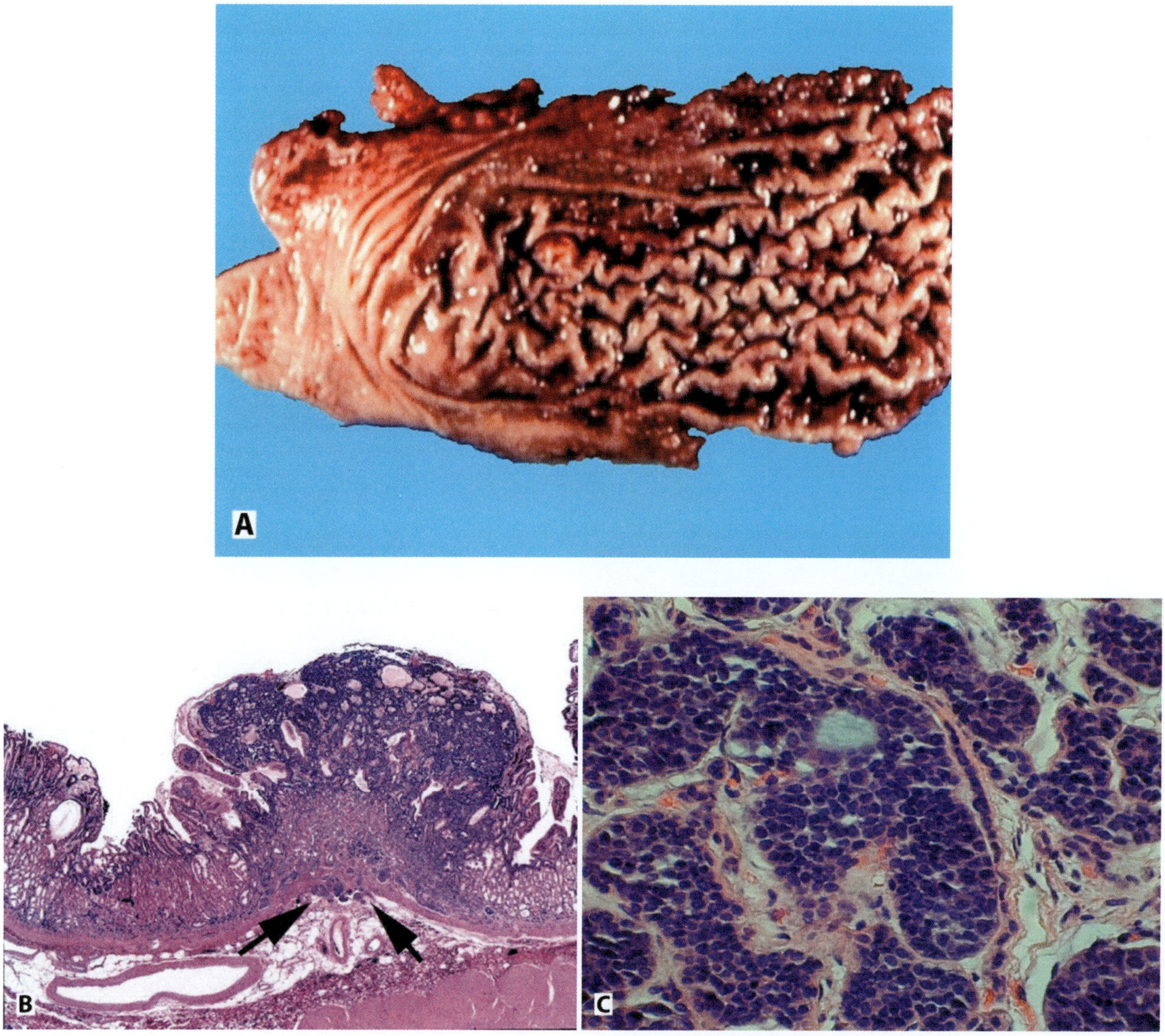

Figure. 3.1 Multiple neuroendocrine tumors: (A) multiple small nodules of carcinoid tumor over mucosa of resected stomach (B) one of the tumors of stomach showing infiltration in submucosa (arrows) (C) high magnification of small round cells arranged in solid nests separated by delicate stroma

Carcinoid tumors (NETs) of small intestine (including duodenum)

(Figure. 3.2)

Definition

Endocrine tumors of small intestine reveal differences according to the anatomical site and type specific endocrine cells involved in tumor formation (Table 3.3): classification of gastroenteropancreatic tumors: (5))

The basic morphology and grading will be similar or common to all types of functioning or non- functioning neuroendocrine tumors of duodenum, jejunum and ileum Table 3.4 (5).

Duodenal Neuroendocrine Tumors

These include gastrinoma, somatostatinoma, serotonin secreting tumor, VIPoma and Gangliocytic paraganglioma..

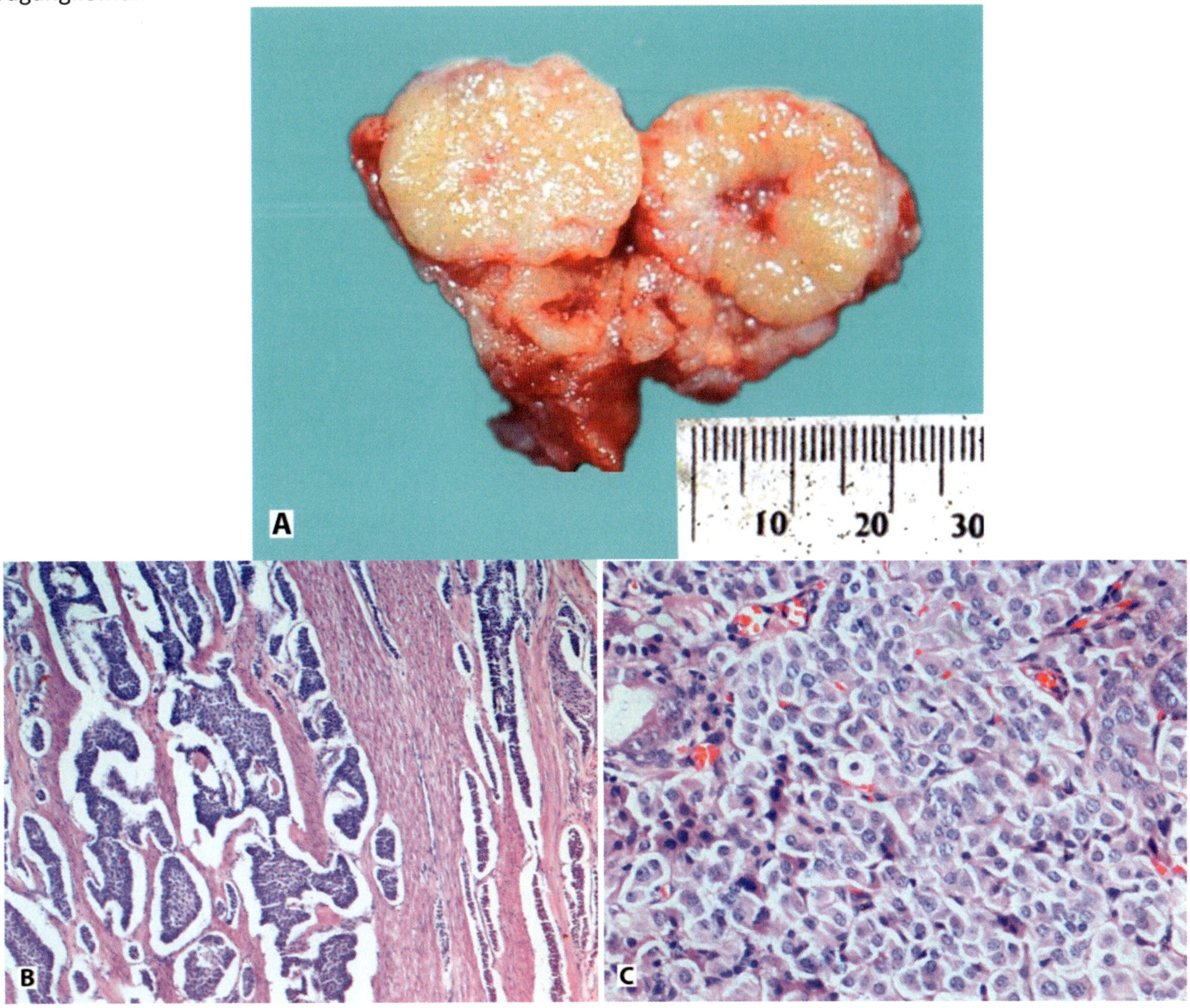

Figure 3.2 Carcinoid tumor of duodenum (non-functioning): (A) a 2 cm yellowish white nodule occupying submucosa and muscularis (B) islands of small cells infiltrating deep into muscularis (C) sheets of neuroendocrine cells containing round pale staining nuclei with fine chromatin

Clinical findings:

The presenting features include bleeding, polypoid mucosal growth, excess hormone induced symptoms (gastrinoma, Somatostatinoma, carcinoid syndrome), jaundice (ampullary tumors) and in few cases symptoms of associated neurofibromatosis (NF 1).

Gastrin-Producing (G cell) neuroendocrine tumors (Gastrinoma)

This is the most frequent subtype of duodenal NET, accounting for over 60% of NETs at this site. About 30% exhibit lymph node metastasis. Generally all hormone secreting endocrine tumors are mostly low grade malignant tumors. Gastrinoma, not infrequently, is encountered in a syndrome of multiple endocrine neoplasia (MEN 1) (12, 16). The subject of gastrinoma is further described in detail in the section on pancreatic neuroendocrine tumors (NETs)

Somatostatin-Producing (D cell) NET

This lesion is characterized by its frequent occurrence in periampullary region, association with von Recklinghausen syndrome in 30% of cases, and presence of pseudo acini with psammoma bodies histologically (Figure. 3.3). It has been commonly misdiagnosed as adenocarcinoma. The symptoms induced by somatostatin hormone are not dramatic or readily diagnostic. The patients display moderate hyperglycemia, cholelithiasis and constipation. Dayal and others compared duodenal carcinoids from patient with and without associated neurofibromatosis and found that 8 of 9 carcinoids with associated VR disease were pure somatostatinomas. (17, 18)

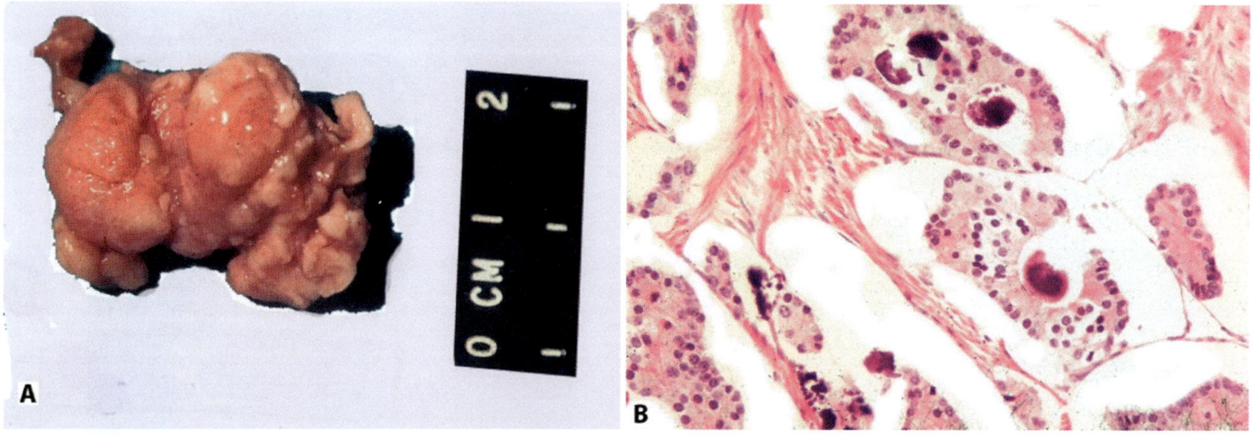

Figure. 3.3 (A) nodule < 1cm in periampullary pancreatic tissue (B) presence of pseudoacini with psammoma bodies can be mistaken as adenocarcinoma

Serotonin-Producing NET

This is the classical carcinoid tumor characterized by no known predisposing condition, nested growth pattern and serotonin secretions. It may metastasize to liver and give rise to typical carcinoid syndrome. (18, 19)

Gangliocytic Paraganglioma

(Figure. 3.4 A-G)

This unique neuroendocrine tumor arises almost exclusively in the II part of the duodenum and particularly in ampullary region. The lesion is typically submucosal, nodular, polypoid, 2-4 cm in size and may cause obstructive jaundice. The tumor exhibits differentiation in different cell types including epithelioid cells in nests and trabeculae, spindle cells in fascicles and scattered ganglion cells. It will variously stain with chromogranin A, synaptophysin, NSE, somatostatin and pancreatic peptide hormones.

The Gangliocytic paragangliomas behave in a benign fashion but lymph node metastasis is encountered in few cases. A recent large epidemiological survey of 192 GP cases published in literature worldwide has produced valuable data, which is as follows: in 173 of 192 (69%) the tumor involved duodenum and lymph node metastasis was found in 12 of 173 (6.9%) cases. The tumor was larger in size and occurred in younger patients with lymph node metastasis (20, 21,22)

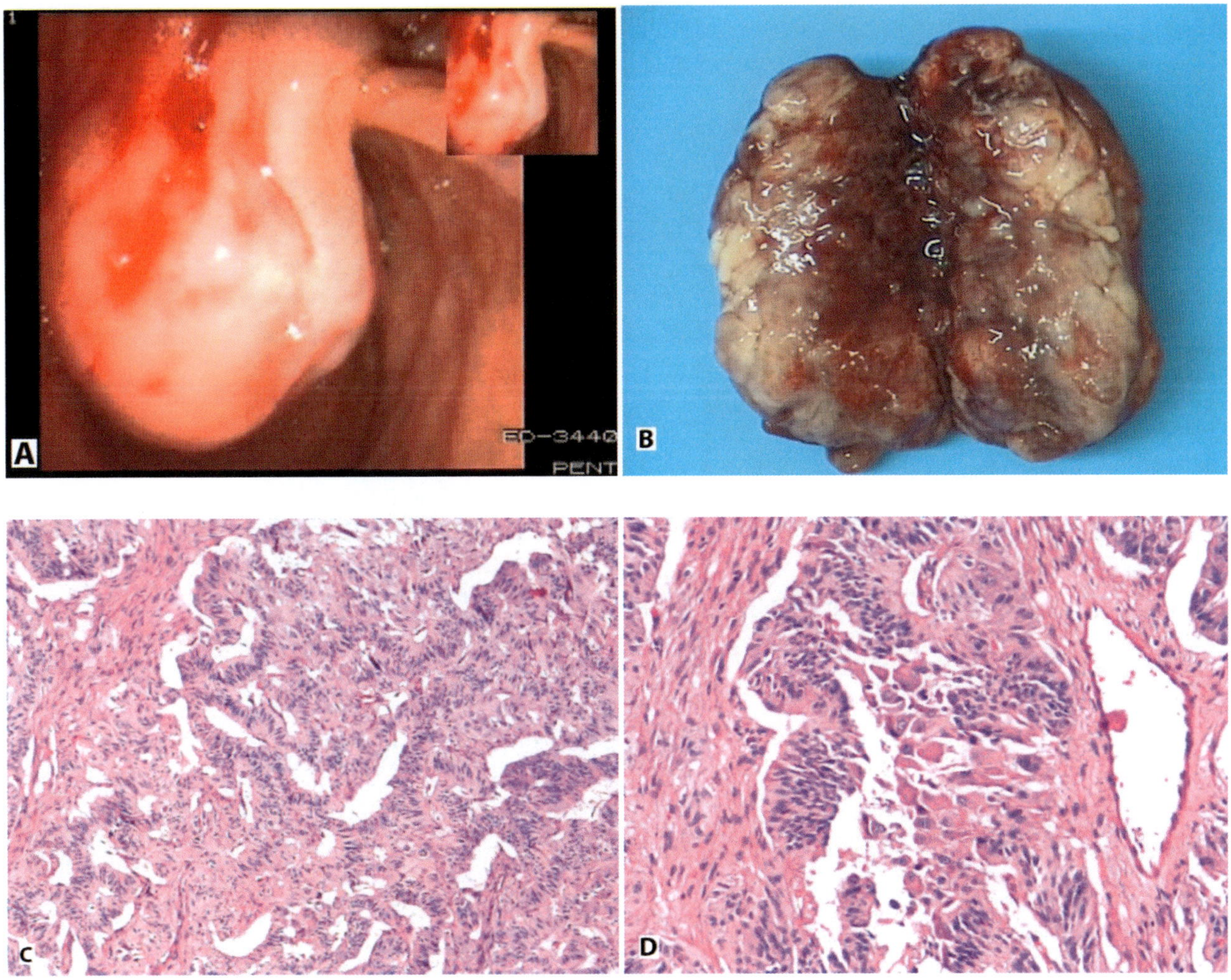

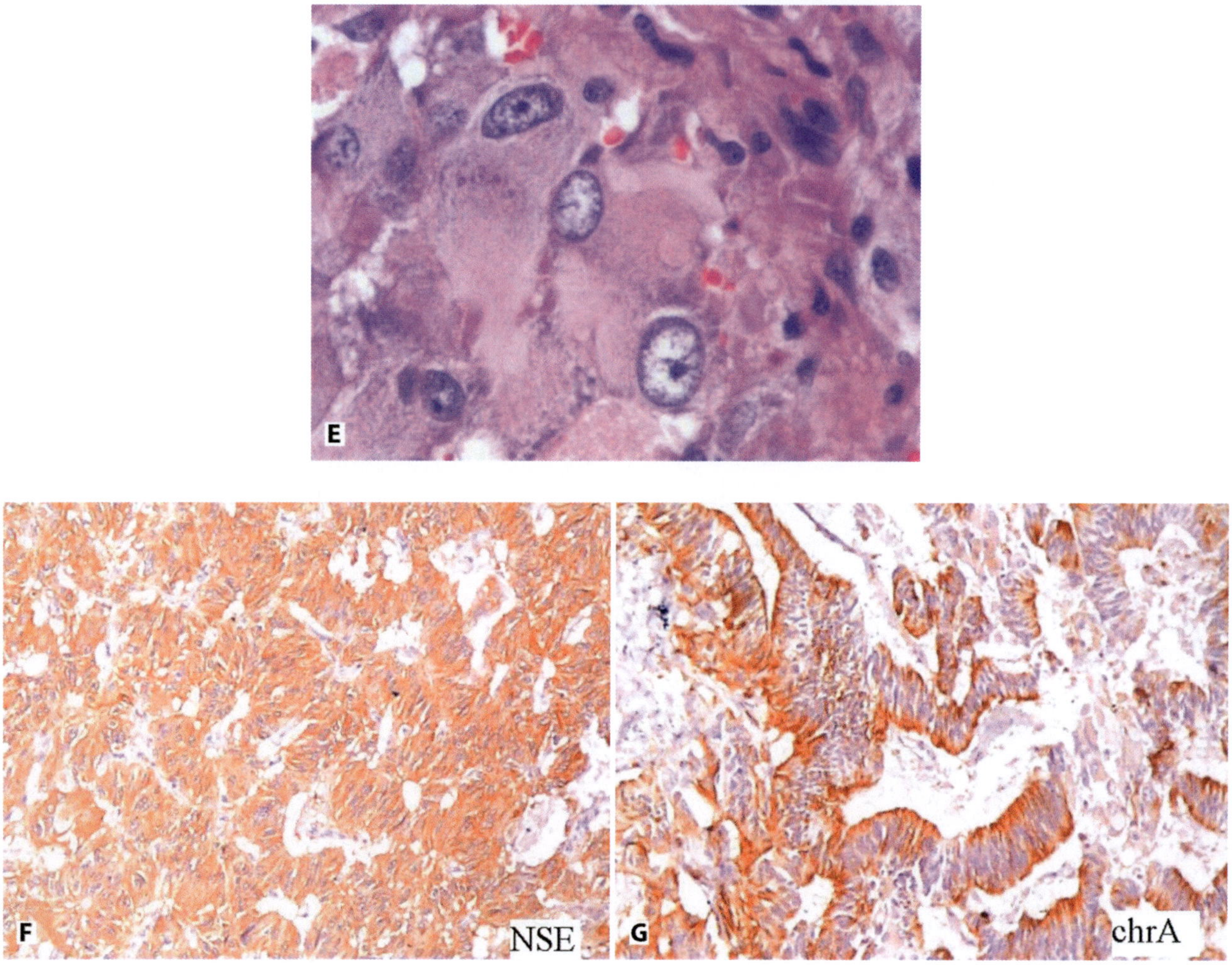

Figure 3.4 Gangliocytic Paraganglioma (A) smooth polypoid mass on endoscopy; (B) bisected tumor, (C, D) epithelioid and trabecular pattern (E) note large ganglion cells (F) strongly positive NSE (G) chromogranin focal strong staining. (Curtsey Dr Anita Shah, Pathologist Breach Candy Hospital)

Jejunal/Ileal Neuroendocrine tumors

NETs in jejunum and ileum are the most common (42%) among all GI NETs and at the time of clinical diagnosis the tumors were larger than 2 cm and showed transmural infiltration and metastasis in lymph nodes and liver.

Clinical Findings

Abdominal pain, nausea, vomiting and weight loss are the most frequent presenting symptoms. Signs of intestinal obstruction occur in some cases, usually secondary to ischemia related fibrosis and elastosis in the adventitia along with marked narrowing of medium sized vessels. Not uncommonly, diagnosis of small bowel NET is made because of the presence of carcinoid syndrome with elevated levels of serum 5 HIAA. Serotonin producing tumors constitute most of the small bowel carcinoids and majority of carcinoid syndrome cases arise in small bowel.

Pathological Features

Small intestinal NETs occur as firm nodules just below the mucosal surface or within intestinal wall or bulge into mucosa. The size varies from 1 to 2 cm and can be as large as 3.5 cm. It appears pale brown or tan yellow on cut section. Histologically, the tumor cells appear small round or cuboidal forming nests separated by delicate vascular strands. The nuclei have fine stippled chromatin and indistinct nucleoli. A trabecular or acinar pattern may be encountered. There is a variable desmoplasia, often quite marked with sclerosing elastotic change in adventitia and intima of medium sized mesenteric arteries. Fibrosis involves muscle and serosa, which can cause kinking of the bowel loop leading to obstruction. Local lymph nodes are involved early and metastatic tumor bearing nodes may be larger than the primary growth. Hepatic metastases are common and can be quite massive, which may be the presenting feature without known prior intestinal carcinoid.

Prognosis

At the time of the clinical diagnosis, 60% of small intestinal carcinoids show metastasis to nodes. Even a small sized (<1 cm) NET can metastasize and cause death. Hence, small intestinal carcinoid is to be considered a potentially malignant lesion. However, these tumors exhibit a characteristic slow indolent growth and 5 year survival of 40% to 58% is far better than 5% survival rate of stage matched adenocarcinoma. A long term survival in patients with hepatic metastases has been reported. In a study of 167 jejunal-ileal 121 NETs 5% had carcinoid syndrome, 26% were multiple, 77% murally invasive, 31% had nodal metastasis and 5 year survival was 58% (23). In the last 3 decades no change has been seen in the mortality of ileal carcinoids (24,25). The salient points about diagnosis of malignant carcinoid tumor include cellular pleomorphism, size >2 cm, irregular hyperchromatic nuclei, frequent mitotic activity, necrosis, invasion muscularis mucosae.

Colonic Neuroendocrine Tumor

(Recto-sigmoid and Appendix excluded)

Majority of colonic NETs arise from, enterochromaffin cells and a few are undifferentiated small cell carcinomas similar to "oat" cell carcinoma of lung, Colonic carcinoids are the most aggressive and clinically present with abdominal mass, weight loss and dyspeptic symptoms.

At surgery the tumors are found to be large, bulky and invasive. Only 5% of these cases exhibit carcinoid syndrome and 65% occur in cecum and right colon. In an epidemiological study of 279 cases 203 were colonic and 76 ileo-cecal carcinoid tumors. The characteristic features included high incidence in females, cecum very commonly involved, 90% cases had >2 cm tumor size, delay in detection of right colonic site tumors, 61% with metastases at detection and 5 year survival about 40%. The 5- year survival rate was only 25% for those with distant spread. (26, 27, 28, 29)

Recto-sigmoid Neuroendocrine Tumor

Rectal carcinoids account for 27% of all GI carcinoids. In a recent series, carcinoids of midgut (cecum to transverse colon) represented about 8% and those of hindgut (descending colon to recto-sigmoid) 20% of total 5973 gastrointestinal carcinoids. It is a slow growing tumor with a low incidence (14%) of lymph node metastasis. Rectal carcinoids are almost never associated with the carcinoid syndrome. The lesion is a sessile polyp or a small (<1 cm) nodule with yellowish cut surface and located in the mid-portion of the rectum. About 50% of rectal carcinoids are asymptomatic and discovered on rectal examination and endoscopy. The remaining 50% give rise to rectal bleeding, pain and constipation. Rectal carcinoids secrete a variety of peptide hormones including enteroglucagon (glycentin), PYY and pancreatic polypeptide. However, unlike other carcinoids rectal NET does not secrete chromogranin A but in its place chromogranin B is identified immunohistochemically. Whereas, a vast majority of these carcinoids are adequately treated with local excision radical surgery is carried out in case of large sized (>2 cm) tumor with muscle invasion, necrosis and high mitotic rate. The 5 year survival is a robust 88% and occurrence of invasion and metastasis is as low as 4%. In one study, malignant carcinoids accounted for 71% of colonic carcinoids and only 14% cases among rectal carcinoids. (30, 31, 32, 33, 34)

Appendicular Neuroendocrine Tumor

Most appendicular carcinoids are removed incidentally at laparotomy and some removed with a prior diagnosis of acute appendicitis. They are usually small, rarely metastasize and usually do not give rise to carcinoid syndrome. A few may behave in a malignant fashion and this is often apparent at laparotomy. There are three major histological types of neuroendocrine tumors: conventional EC cell tumor, goblet cell carcinoid and L-cell NET. Of these, EC cell tumor is the most frequent and well-studied NET, 70% occurring at the tip (Figure. 3.5 A-D) and 20% in the mid portion. They are pale yellow colored <1 cm nodules typically arising from the submucosa, although invasion in muscularis and lymphatics is quite common. (35, 36, 37)

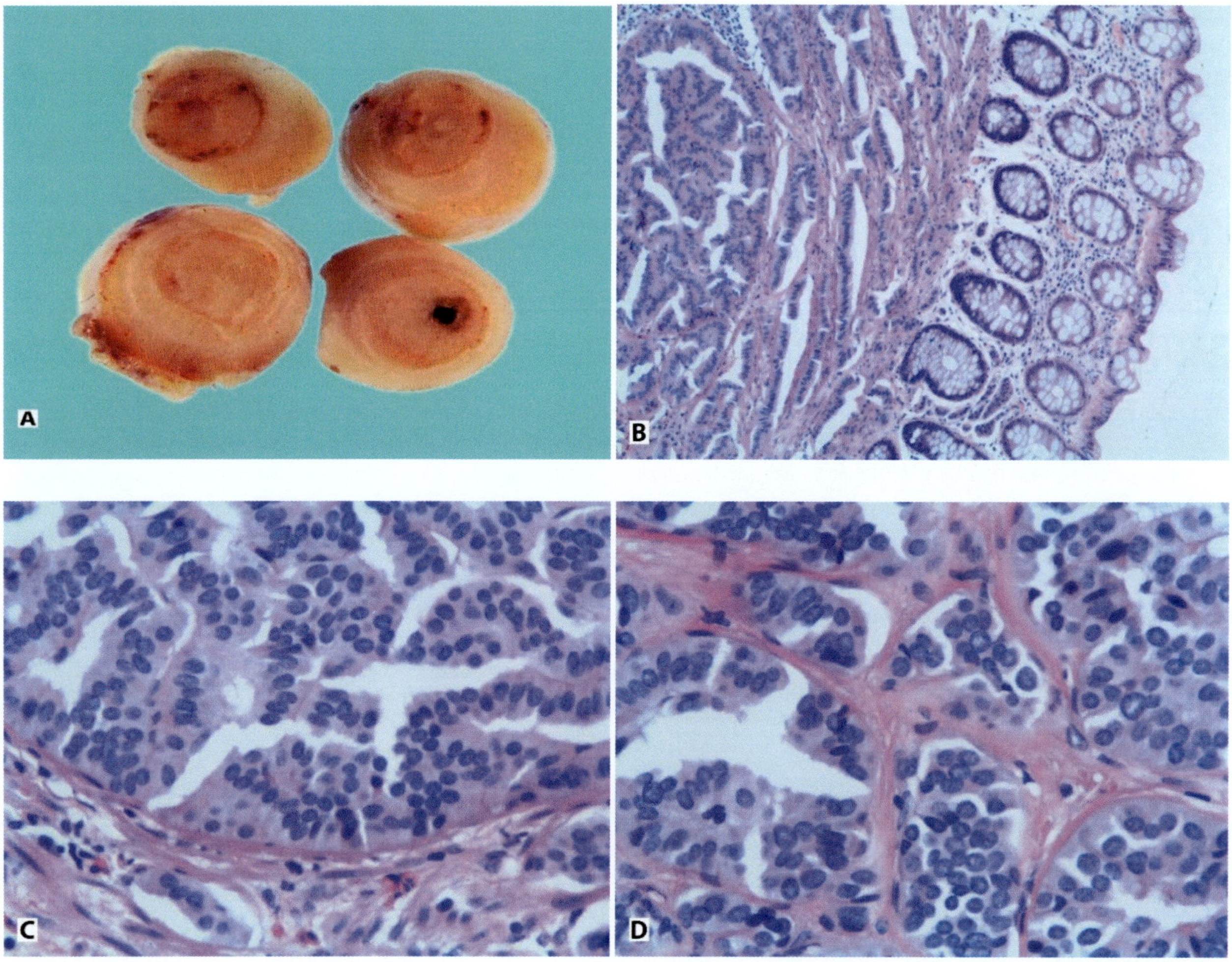

Figure 3.5 Carcinoid of appendix: (A) transverse section of thick swollen appendix plugged with pale tan yellowish tumor (B) intact appendicular mucosa overlying the tumor having trabecular pattern (C, D) small, uniform oval to round nuclei without anaplasia

Goblet cell carcinoid involves the appendix almost exclusively and the term goblet cell carcinoid has many synonyms: adenocarcinoid, mucinous carcinoid, crypt cell carcinoid and mucin producing neuroendocrine tumor.

This unique tumor arises from pluripotent crypt-base stem cells and shows dual differentiation, neuroendocrine and mucinous. Goblet cell carcinoid (GCC) is composed of mixture of normal crypt cells, goblet cells, Paneth cells and also enterochromaffin cells. The histological hallmark is the presence of clusters of goblet cells in the lamina propria or submucosa, and stain with neuroendocrine markers with patchy intensity (Figure 3.6

A, B, C). The tumor typically shows glandular collections of cells distended with mucous giving resemblance to goblet cells or signet ring cells (Figure. 3.6 A). Endocrine cells are sparsely populated and typically contain small peripheral nuclei with no pleomorphism and no mitotic activity. Size of the tumor and perineural lymphatic spread are unreliable prognostic features in GCC.

The prognosis of GCC is intermediate between appendicular carcinoid and pure appendicular adenocarcinoma. However, a subset of GCC is particularly aggressive. These reveal a mixture of conventional goblet cell carcinoid and foci of pure adenocarcinoma or typical signet ring cells with prominent nuclear anaplasia. The goblet cell carcinoid is known to metastasize to the ovary with no clinical evidence of appendiceal tumor. The ovarian tumor is often bilateral and is diagnosed as primary mucinous tumors of ovary (38, 39, 40, 41).

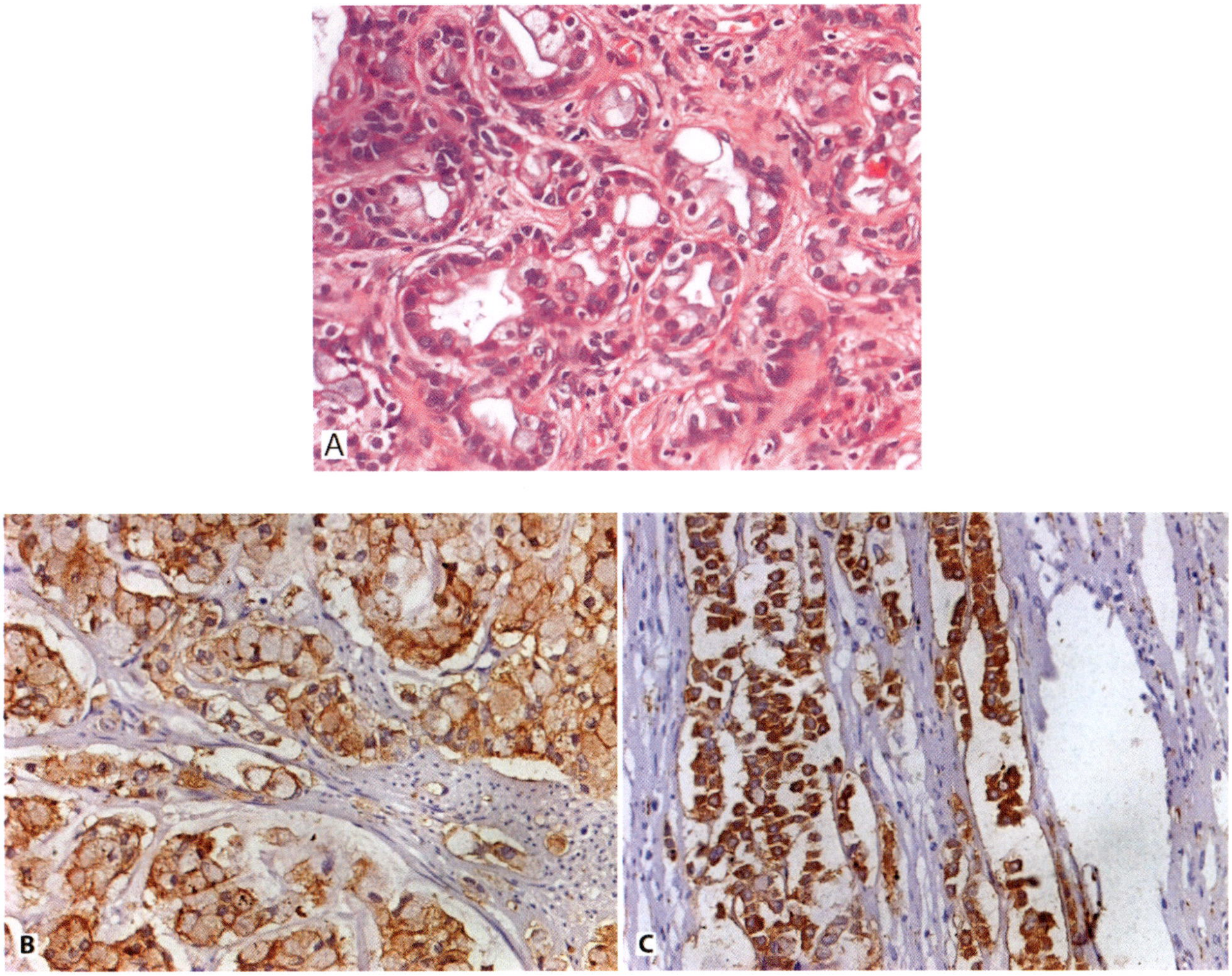

Figure 3.6 Goblet cell carcinoid (A) many cuboidal cells filled mucin and scattered small round cells (B) synaptophysin staining the mucinous cells (C) synaptophysin staining the small cell component

L-cell NET of Appendix

This type of NET is quite uncommon, very small (2-3 mm) in size and express enteroglucagon, PYY and pancreatic polypeptide but no chromogranin A. They are composed of small acini or tubules dispersed in loose fibrous stroma. The prognosis is good and some believe that they may not be truly neoplastic and represent a reactive change (37).

Treatment

Simple appendectomy is adequate and curative for appendiceal carcinoid <1 cm. For tumors 1-2 cm a simple appendectomy followed by periodic follow up for 5 years is recommended. Right hemicolectomy, 3 months after appendectomy, should be reserved for tumors >2 cm, tumor at the base of appendix, cecal infiltration, invasion into mesoappendix and associated adenocarcinoma.(42)

Pancreatic Endocrine Tumors (PETs):

General Considerations

(43, 44, 45, 46)

A variety of functionally active endocrine tumors occurs in pancreas and these give rise to very dramatic signs and symptoms, which are typical of many clinical syndromes. All pancreatic endocrine tumors secrete a multitude of peptic hormones and amines, which cause clinical syndromes: insulin syndrome, glucagonoma syndrome, Zollinger-Ellison syndrome (excess gastrin secretions), VIPOMAS and WHDA (watery diarrhea, hypocalcemia and achlorhydria). This has been also called as Verner-Morrison syndrome. The tumors are quite uncommon but their incidence has been increasing in the recent years. This is apparently due to application of more sensitive diagnostic approaches such as: imaging techniques, reliable laboratory tests and analysis by immunohistochemical and molecular biology assays. The relative incidence of PETs from the WHO data is given in Table 3.7. Tables 3.8, 3.9 show the author's experience of various pancreatic lesions, including the list of 21 endocrine tumors (incidence 2.3%).

Pancreatic Endocrine Tumors

(WHO data: n=638, Heitz PU, Bordi C, Komminath P,et al. WHO classification of Tumors, Pathology and Genetics : Tumors of Endocrine Organs. Delellis PA, Lloyd RV, Heitz PU, Eng C (Eds) IARC press Lyon, 2004) (45)

Table 3.7 : Pancreatic Endocrine Tumors (WHO data: n=638)*	
Insulinomas	174(27.2%)
Gastrinomas	80(12.5%)
Glucagonomas	51 (8%)
VIPomas	41 (6.4%) 24
Somatostatinoma	24 (3.80%)
Ectopic hormone tumors	15(2.4%
Nonfunctioning	253 (39.7%)

*Heitz PU, Bordi C, Komminath P,et al. WHO classification of Tumors, Pathology and Genetics : Tumors of Endocrine Organs. Delellis PA, Lloyd RV, Heitz PU, Eng C (Eds) IARC press Lyon, 2004)

Table 3.8: Lesions of Pancreas, n=895 Author's series (1970-2000)	
Adenocarcinoma of pancreas	157
Adenocarcinoma of ampulla	110
Adenoma, cystadenoma	9
Endocrine tumors	21
Non-neoplastic lesions	598
Total	895

Table 3.9: Endocrine tumors of pancreas Author's seris (1970-2000) n=21	
Benign Insulinoma	8
Malignant Insulinoma	2
Malignant Gastrinoma	2
Stomatostatinoma	1
Glucagonoma	1
Carcinoid with syndrome	1
Nonfunctiomng, Benign	4
Nonfunctiomng, malignant	2

Histology:

Most PETs are well differentiated and have different morphological patterns, namely: trabecular, solid, glandular, gyriform, etc. The cells are small to medium sized with pale cytoplasm and finely distributed chromatin ("salt & pepper" nuclei). All features area sufficiently distinctive to permit identification of endocrine nature of a given tumor. In general, histological pattern is not specific for different syndromic tumors and the diagnosis in most instances is made before surgery. There are two exceptions to this rule: amyloid deposit in the tumor is indicative of insulinoma and glandular structures with psammoma bodies are commonly observed in somatostatinoma.

Prediction of the behavior of PETs

The behavior of PETs is difficult to predict on their histological features alone. Metastasis is generally accepted to be the only definitive feature of malignancy. However, several characteristics such as tumor size, presence and type of hyper functioning syndrome, number of mitoses, Ki 67 Proliferative Index, vascular/perineural invasion, necrosis and grade of tumor have been reported as reliable prognostic markers. Multivariate approaches, such as Capella (46) classification combine some of these parameters to group PETs into four subgroups: benign, borderline, low grade malignant and high grade malignant. This classification is based on tumor size, histologic parameters, including tumor differentiation, vascular invasion and functional lineage (46).

Facts:

Insulinomas and nonfunctional noninvasive well differentiated PETs less than 2 cm size usually behave benign.

Insulinomas and nonfunctional tumors greater than 3 cm and /or angioinvasive tumors are generally classified as low grade malignant PETs.

Noninvasive tumors between 2cm and 3cm form a group whose behavior is difficult to predict and are designated as "borderline".

Gastrinoma, VIPoma, glucagonoma, or tumors with Cushing or carcinoid syndromes with >2 cm size and/or angioinvasion are classified as low grade malignant, those less than 1 cm as benign, those between 1 cm and 2 cm as borderline.

Tumors histologically resembling small cell adenocarcinomas constitute the poorly differentiated endocrine carcinomas.

Recently Cytokeratin 19 has been shown to be a powerful predictor of survival in pancreatic endocrine tumors. The authors of this article suggested that all PETs with any one of the following features be diagnosed as malignant: presence of necrosis, vascular invasion, perineurial invasion or CK 19 positivity (47). It is necessary to stain endothelial cells by immunohistochemical marker CD34 to identify small vascular channels, not clearly evident on H & E stain.

Neurofibromatosis & PETs

It is well known that patients with von Recklinghausen syndrome (NF1) are predisposed to endocrine tumors including pheochromocytoma and duodenal neuroendocrine tumors (carcinoids) secreting somatostatin. It is not known whether rarely occurring insulinoma in VRS is an incidental finding or whether it is a rare manifestation of NF1.

Insulinoma, Glucagonoma, Gastrinoma and Somatostatinoma will be described and illustrated.

Insulinoma

(48, 49, 50)

This is insulin secreting common benign endocrine tumor of the Beta cells of islets of Langerhans, giving rise to sustained intractable hypoglycemia before surgical intervention. A vast majority of insulinomas are located in the pancreas and less than 2% in the duodenal wall. The tumors are almost equally distributed in head, body and tail of the pancreas. Determination of plasma insulin and proinsulin concentration by radioimmunoassay has greatly facilitated the diagnosis. Grossly, the tumor is well circumscribed or encapsulated and the malignant ones appear nodular. Microscopic study shows four types of patterns, the most common being trabecular. The cells frequently show bland cytology with no nuclear anaplasia (Figure. 3.7 A-E). One of the most characteristic finding in insulinoma is amyloid stroma. (Figure. 3.7 F, G). Histopathologic study is required mainly to confirm benignancy, which is present in 95% of cases and to look for signs of malignancy such as local invasion and metastasis. Malignant insulinomas may show invasion in the peripancreatic tissue or adjacent organs, and metastases to regional lymph nodes (peripancreatic, celiac and paraaortic) and liver.

The natural history and survival:

A study of 1067 cases of Insulinoma (Stephanini P, Carboni M, Pathrossi N, et al. Beta islet cell tumors of the pancreas: results of a study of 1067 cases. Surgery 1974; 75:597-609) (49)

638/1012 (63%) completely documented cases were reported to be all cured. In 772 (76%) cases tumor was found at operation. In 74 (7%) cases no tumor was found at operation. Second operation was required in 111 (11%) cases, multiple operations were required in 58 (5.7%) cases. The distribution of tumors was as follows: head (305), body (285) & tail (323). In 789 (83%) cases single tumor present, in 123 (13%) cases multiple tumors present and 39 (4%) cases were associated with MEN 1. Different types of surgeries included: enucleation 506 (50%), distal resection 415(41%), subtotal resection 20 (2%) and pancreatico-duodenectomy 15 (1.5%)

Service FJ, McMahon MM, Obstriet PC, et al Functioning insulinoma: incidence, recurrences and long term survival of patients, 60 year study Mayo Clin Proc 1991; 66:711-719 (50)

Median age in this study was 47 yrs. in males and 59 yrs. in females. Recurrence rate associated with MEN1 was 21% at 10-20 years in contrast to 5% recurrence rate associated with sporadic cases at 10 years & 7% at 20 years. The 10 year survival in cases of benign Insulinoma was 88% vs 29% in cases of malignant insulinomas.

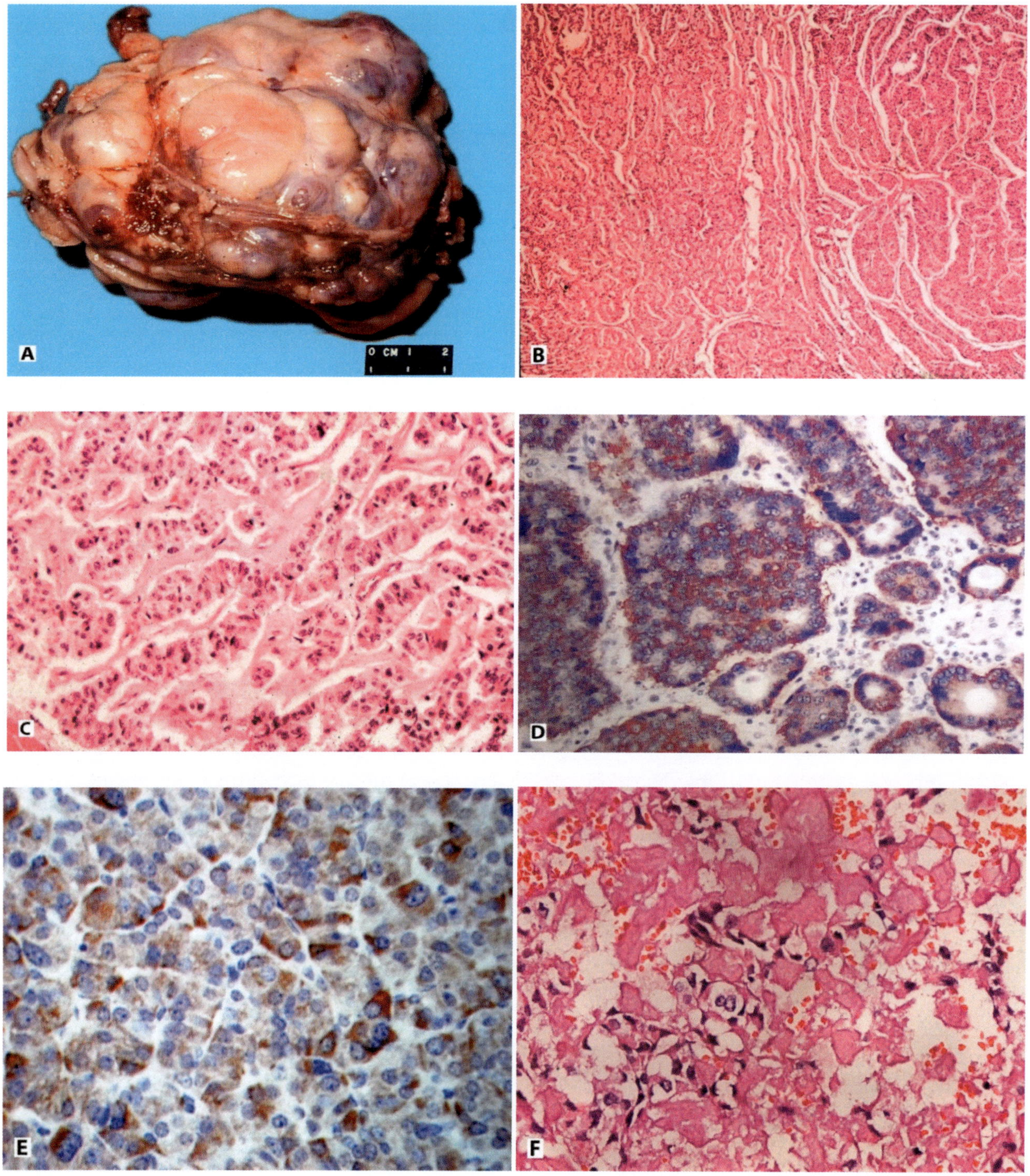

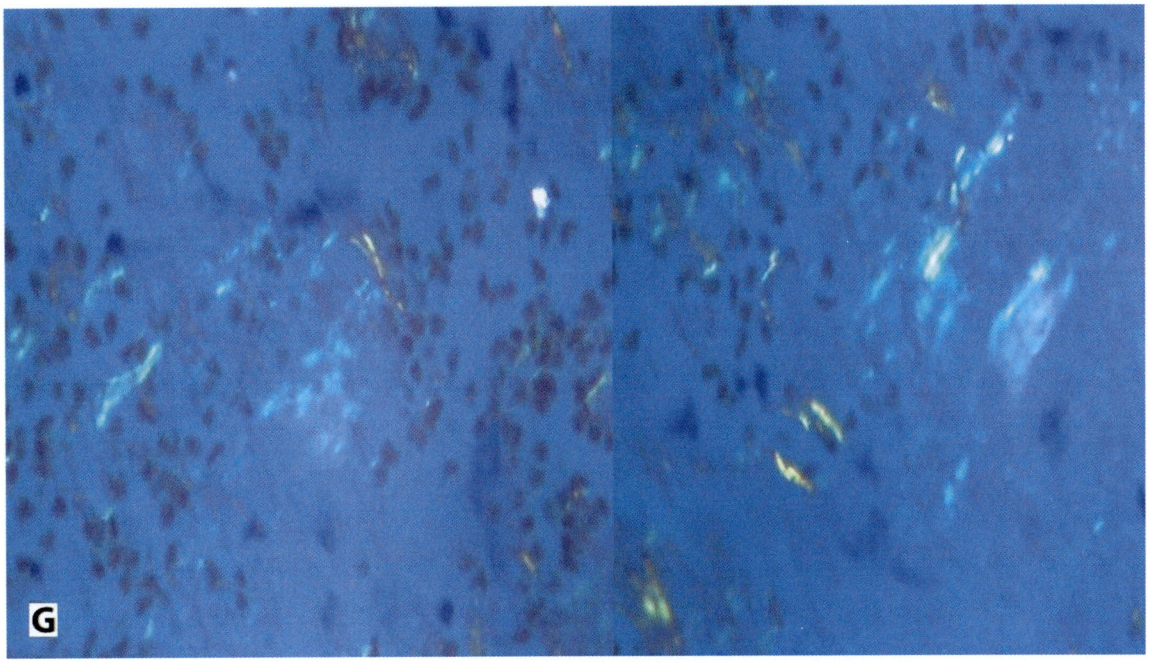

Figure 3.7 Insulinoma of pancreas: (A) non-functioning malignant Insulinoma is a bosselated well encapsulated 11 x 8 x 5 cm mass, (B& C) trabecular pattern; variable nuclear anaplasia (D) glandular pattern (E) tumor cells express insulin on immunohistochemistry (F) histology of amyloid stroma in insulinoma (G) Cong red stain showing focal green fluorescence on polarized light

Glucagonoma

Glucagonoma syndrome is a paraneoplastic phenomenon characterized by islet alpha-cell pancreatic tumor, necrolytic migratory erythema, diabetes mellitus, weight loss, anemia, stomatitis, thromboembolism, gastrointestinal disturbances and neuropsychiatric symptoms. The frequency of each of these presenting signs is shown in Table 3.10. These findings in association with hyperglucagonemia and demonstrable pancreatic tumor establish the diagnosis. Most patients are diagnosed too late in the clinical course for cure but successful palliation of symptomatology can usually be achieved. Glucagonoma associated with MEN 1 syndrome tend to be multiple in about 59% of cases. Majority of glucagonoma are large solitary tumors with a 7 cm mean diameter (Figure. 3.8 A-C). The histological features are not distinctive in any way and the diagnosis is often suggested by a set of presenting symptoms confirmed by demonstration of hyperglucagonemia.

The tumors spread by local invasion into surrounding tissues and metastasize to regional nodes and liver. About 60 % to 70% glucagonomas present with metastasis at the time of diagnosis. Even small sized (<0.5 cm) glucagonomas are known to show uncertain behavior or a histologically identified well differentiated endocrine carcinoma. (51, 52)

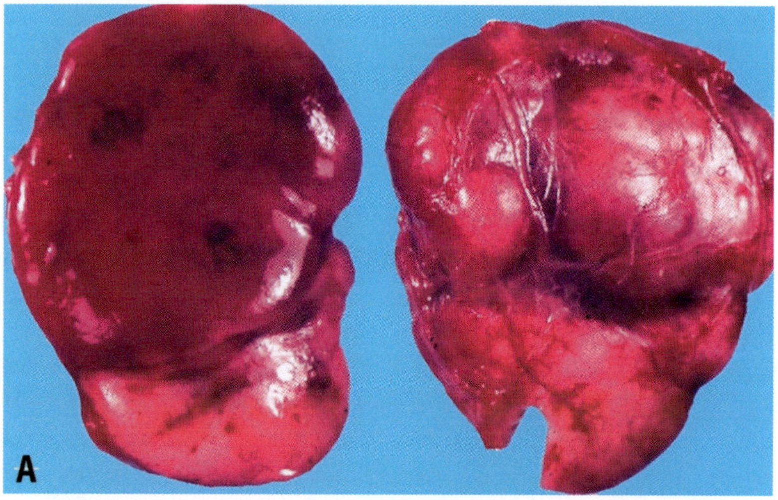

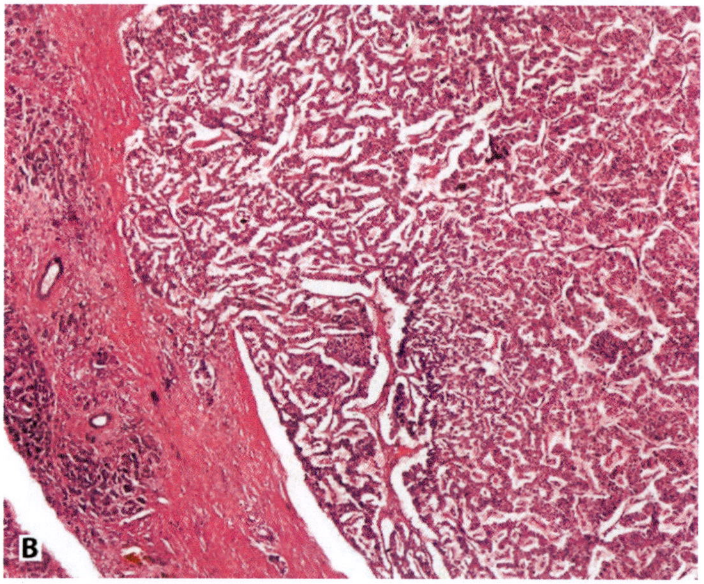

Figure 3.8 Glucagonoma: (A) encapsulated bosselated functioning glucagonoma (B) trabecular pattern of neoplastic endocrine cells and the tumor invading the thick fibrous capsule

Table 3.10 Clinical features of glucagonomas-407 cases	
Associated with MEN1	53/407 (13%)
Incidence of multiple tumors	48/407 (12%)
Situated in tail of pancreas	213/407 (54%)
Malignancy	247/407 (61%)
Metastases	209/407 (51%)
Patients with Diabetico-dermatogenic Syndrome (DDS)	233/407 (57%)
10yr survival in 233 cases with DDS	with metastasis-52% without metastasis 64%

Modified and adaoted from Soga J, Yakuwa Y. Glucagonomas/diabetic-dermatogenic Syndrome: a statistical evaluation of 407 reported cases. J Hepatobiliary Pancreat Surg 1998; 5:312-319 (52)

Gastrinoma

Gastrinomas are gastrin producing endocrine tumors that occur almost exclusively in pancreatico-duodenal region. Most are functional, causing hypergastrinemia and Zollinger Ellison syndrome (ZES). This syndrome is characterized by multiple duodenal peptic ulcers prominent gastric rugal folds secondary to an increased oxyntic gland mass, and steatorrhoea. Two types of gastrinomas occur: sporadic non familial gastrinoma with ZES (80% of cases) and familial gastrinoma with ZES in the setting of MEN 1 (20% of cases). Gastrinomas are relatively common functioning endocrine tumors of pancreas and duodenum and are second in frequency only to insulinomas.

Location of gastrinomas is much more common in pancreas (53%) than in duodenum or jejunum (13%) according to the data of ZES tumor registry with 800 cases as of 1973 (53).

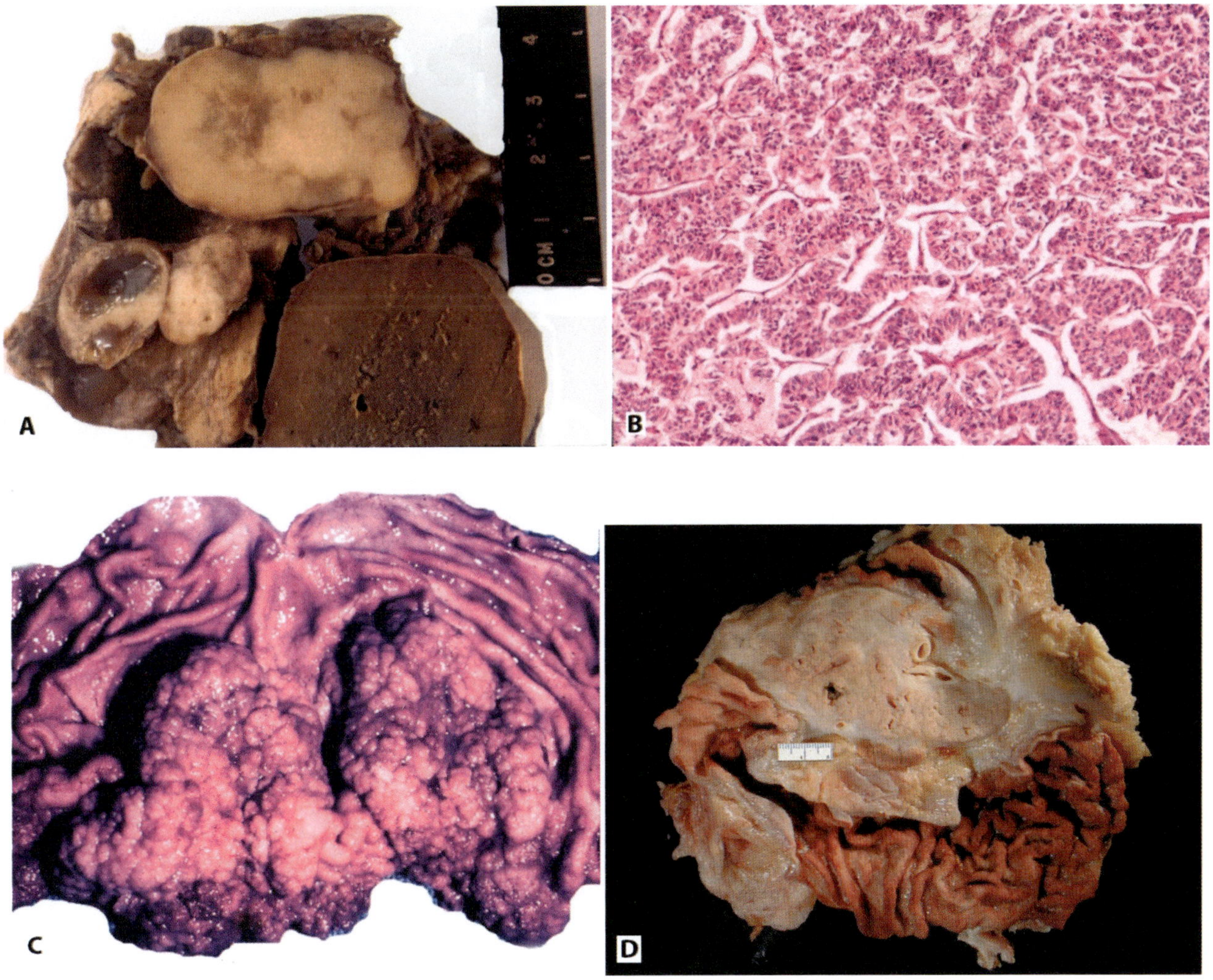

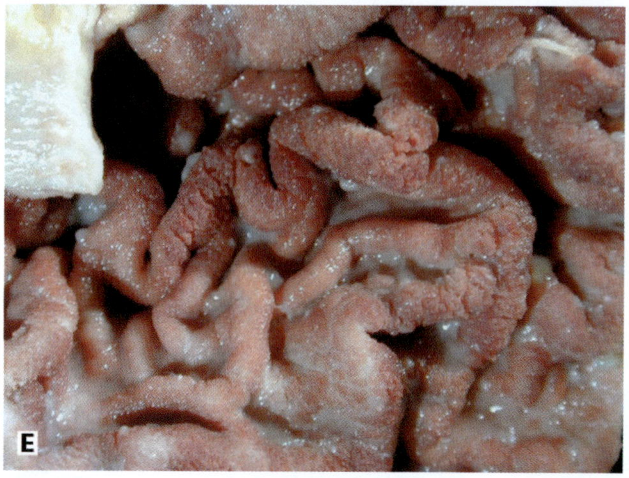

Figure 3.9 Zollinger–Ellison syndrome: (A) A large 6 cm encapsulated tumor with satellite nodules and spleen with stomach in the background (B) typical trabecular pattern of a cellular lesion (C) gastric mucosal folds (rugae) enormously thickened due to florid hyperplasia of parietal cells, superficially resembling a neoplasm, no adenoma, was found. (D) ill-defined tumor in pancreas adherent to stomach (E) hypertrophic gastric mucosal rugae

Gastrinoma are usually residing within "gastrinoma triangle", which is formed by junction of cystic duct and common duct, the junction of II and III parts of duodenum and junction of neck and body of the pancreas. It is extraordinary that gastrinoma has been reported in far flung organ systems including stomach, biliary tract, liver, kidney, mesentery and heart.

Gastrinomas are cellular tumors (Figure. 3.9 A-E) composed of anastomosing cords, trabeculae and lobules lined by monotonous cells with eosinophilic cytoplasm and round nuclei having fine chromatin. Both sporadic gastrinomas and those associated with the setting of MEN 1 may be multifocal. Multiple sporadic gastrinomas probably represent metastasis, because all independent tumors share identical mutations and other genetic changes. Those associated with MEN 1 have varied genetic abnormalities and probably represent independent primary tumors. It is important to distinguish gastrinomas from other type of PETs because gastrinoma diagnosis has far reaching clinical implications. Incidentally discovered duodenal lesions associated with chronic acid suppression or gastritis, behave in a clinically indolent fashion and should be treated conservatively. Peripancreatic and periduodenal gastrinomas are thought to represent primary tumors rather than metastases from an occult primary in the duodenum. Some patients have been cured after resection of the tumorous nodes.

Treatment & Prognosis

Management of ZES is a formidable problem because of dreadful consequences of acid overproduction, difficulty in localizing of gastrinoma particularly in the duodenum (often small sized), multiple tumors and overall poor survival. The use of powerful acid anti secretory agents like H2 receptor antagonist and proton pump inhibitors has profoundly facilitated management of ZES. In the past patients with ZES were treated with total gastrectomy but now the care is primarily focused on management of the gastrinoma tumor (54, 55).

A series of 52 cases of ZES a search for gastrinomas was carried out at exploratory laparotomy.

The study gives a wealth of information about the role of surgery in the management and its effects on prognosis (54).

Gastrinoma involves the entire pancreas in most patients with MEN 1

Total pancreatectomy may be necessary to cure ZES in MEN 1

It is possible to cure some patients with hepatic metastases

Tumors of the head of pancreas can be cured by enucleation alone

The morbidity of operations aimed at removing all gastrinoma is very low today.

Resections of all visible gastrinomas in patient without MEN have about 70% chance of curing the patient.

The quality of life after successful surgery is so much better than other forms of therapy that possibility of resection should be aggressively pursued in every patient

Gastrinoma in patients with liver metastasis behave more aggressively (55) than those with only lymph node metastasis. In fact lymph node metastases have little or no influence on the survival on patients with ZES (56). The frequency of metastasis is 30% in patients with pancreatic gastrinoma and only 3% in patients with duodenal tumors. Metastases to other organs are indeed rare. It has been observed that duodenal gastrinomas are less malignant (38%) than pancreatic ones (60%). In general progression of gastrinomas is relatively slow with a combined 5-year survival of 65% and 10-year survival of 51%. Even with metastatic disease a 10-year survival for lymph node metastases is 46% and for liver metastases 40%. In patients with complete resection have excellent 5 and 10-year survival rates of 90-100%. Patients with pancreatic tumors have a worst prognosis than those with duodenal tumor: 10-year survival of 9% versus 59%. The rate of death in aggressive forms of gastrinoma ranges from 38% in MEN 1 cases to 62% in sporadic cases. (57, 58, 59, 60)

Nesidioblastosis

(60, 61, 62)

Hyperinsulinism is a rare cause of severe persistent hypoglycemia during the neonatal period. Nevertheless it is a diagnosis of importance since hypoglycemia may be exceedingly difficult to control. The patient should undergo a subtotal pancreatectomy as soon as the diagnosis is reached because of high incidence of brain damage and subsequent mental retardation. The syndrome was described more than 40 years ago but the pathogenesis of the disease has not yet been completely elucidated. The term nesidioblastosis describes the persistence of a diffused disseminated proliferation of islets cells budding off from ducts (ducto-insulinar complex) Electron microscopic study is diagnostic of Nesidioblastosis, in that the characteristic crystalline granules of beta cells can be readily differentiated from zymogen granules (Figures 3.10, 3.11) This excess mass of beta cells is considered to be the underlying cause of the disease. However, it has been seen that nesidioblastosis is encountered in the pancreas in normo-glycemic neonates and infants, which was observed at autopsy. This implies that pathogenesis of nesidioblastosis should be reconsidered and other causative factors be investigated. By means of linkage analysis, hyperinsulinism in familial cases has been shown to chromosome 11 and ongoing genetic studies await the elucidation of the pathogenesis of nesidioblastosis.

Nesidioblastosis is also an infrequent, yet clinically important, cause of hypoglycemia in adult population, and should be considered in a patient with a presumptive diagnosis of insulinoma. A 70% distal pancreatectomy will be successful in controlling hyperglycemia in these patients, and would rarely result in diabetes mellitus (63)

A case of hyperinsulinimic hypoglycemic coma in a 1 year old child is illustrated in (Figures 3.10 & 3.11).

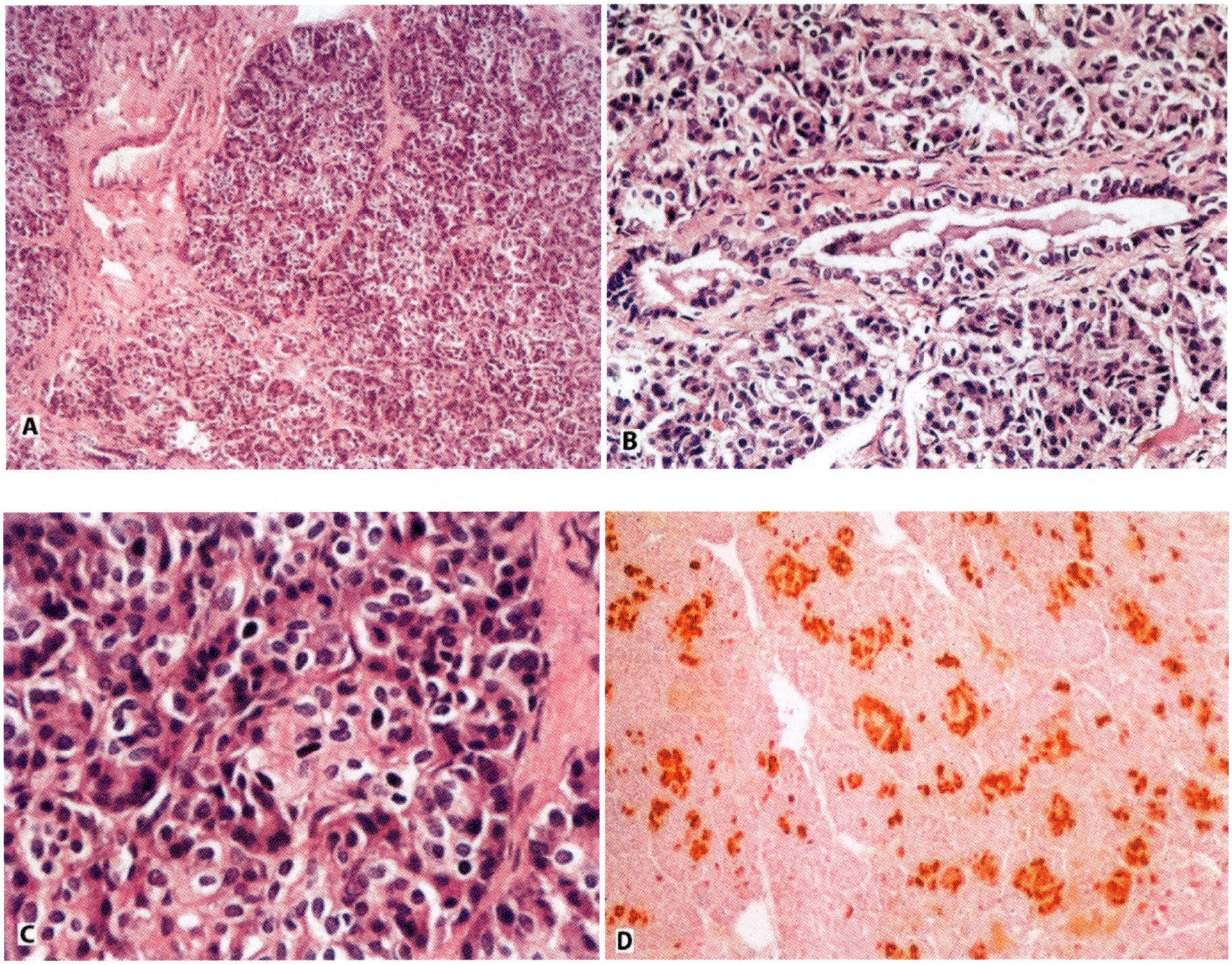

Figure 3.10 Nesidioblastosis (A) Section of pancreas exhibiting a large population of vacuolated cells (endocrine cells)within the acini, note lack of islets (B) The vacuolated cells are also seen within the lining of pancreatic ducts (C) high power view of overwhelming number of larger vacuolated endocrine cells (D) Numerous small clusters of cells expressing insulin on immunohistochemistry

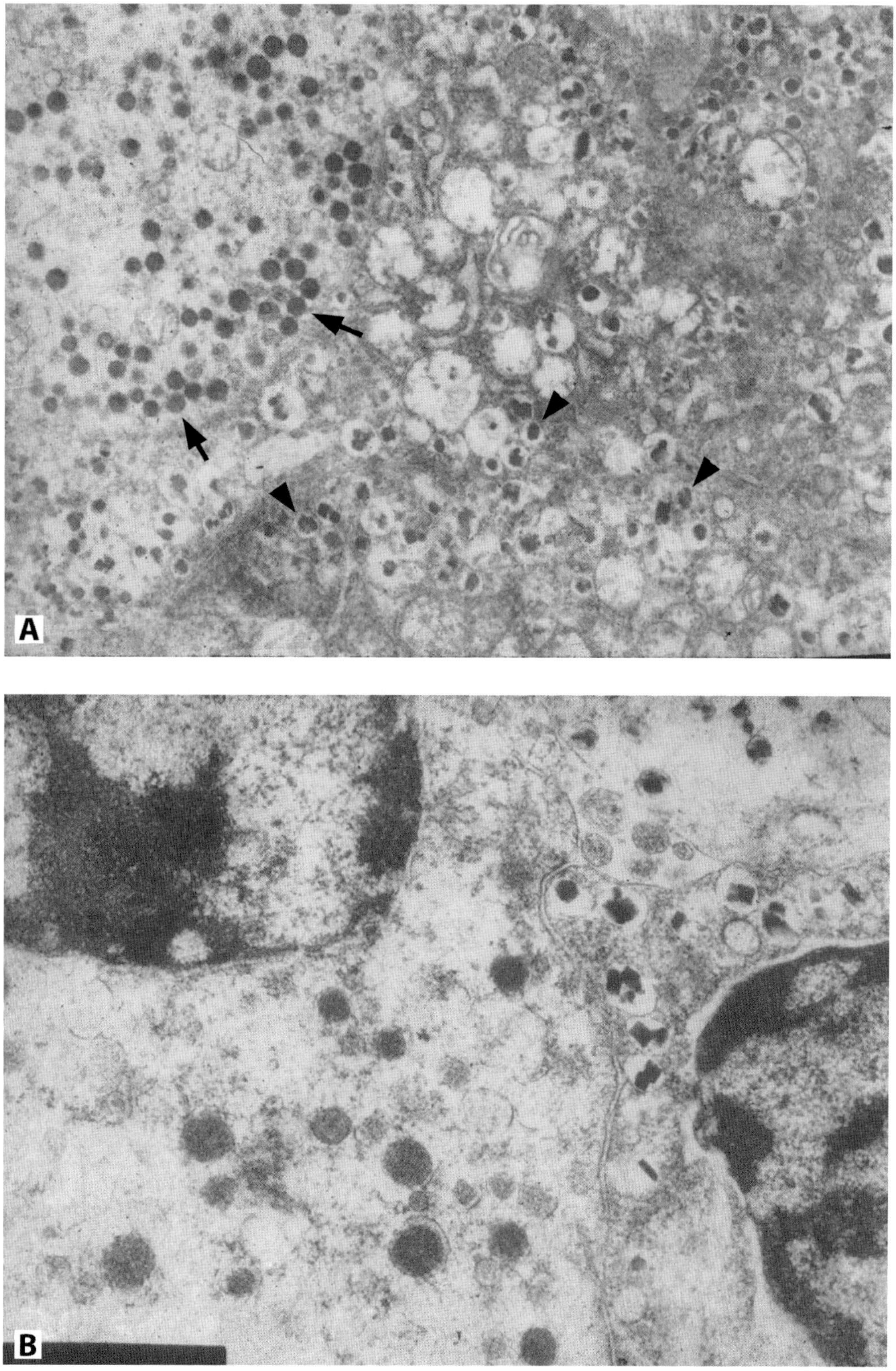

Figure 3.11 (A) Electron microscopy of nesidioblastosis of pancreas: numerous large rounded zymogen granules (black arrows) and irregular pleomorphic beta (insulin) granules (arrow heads)in the same cells (B) higher power shows two cells separated by double plasma membranes with rounded exocrine zymogen granules seen in cell on left and pleomorphic beta insulin granules in cell on right. This is in the same pancreatic acinus.

Refrences of gastro-entero-pancreatic neuroendocrine tumors

1 Kloppel G. Oberndorfer and His Successors: From carcinoid to Neuroendocrine Carcinoma Endocr Pathol 2007; 18:141,

2 Lewin KJ. The endocrine cells of the gastrointestinal tract. The normal endocrine cells and their hyperplasias, Part I. In Sommers Sc, Rosen PP {eds}: Pathology Annual. Part I. Vol 21. Appleton-Century Crafts, East Norwalk, CT, 1986

3 Pearse AGE. The APUD cell concept and its implications in pathology In Sommers Sc {ed}: Pathology Annual. Vol 9. Appleton-Century Crafts/New York, 1974

4 Polak JM and Bloom SR. Neuropeptides of the Gut: A Newly Discovered Major Control System. World J Surg 1979; 3:393

5 Kloppel G, Perren A, Heitz PU: The Gastroenteropancreatic Neuroendocrine Cell System and Its Tumors: The WHO classification. Ann. N. Y. Acad. Sci 2004; 1014:13-27

6 Modlin IM, Lye KD, Kidd M: A 5-decade Analysis of 13,715 Carcinoid Tumors. Cancer 2003; 97: 934-959)

7 Bordi C, D'Adda T, Azzoni C, Ferraro G: Pathogenesis of ECL tumors in humans. Yale J Biol Med. 2003; 71: 273-284)

8 Rindi G, Bordi C, Rappel S, et al: Gastric carcinoids and neuroendocrine carcinomas: Pathogenesis, pathology and behavior. World J Surg 1996; 20: 168-172

9 Bordi C, D'Adda T, Azzoni C, et al: Hypergastrinemia and gastric enterochromaffin-like cases. Am J Surg Pathol 1995; 19(Suppl 1) S8-S19

10 Modlin IM, Lye KD, Kidd M: Carcinoid tumors of the stomach. Surg Oncol 2003; 12: 153-172

11 Modlin IM, Lawton GP, Miu K, et al: Patho-physiology of the fundic enterochromaffin-like{ECL} and gastric carcinoid tumors. Ann R Coll Surg Engl 1996; 78: 1330138

12 Merchant SH, Vanderjagt T, Lathrop S, Amin MB: Sporadic duodenal bulb gastrin-cell tumors: Association with Helicobacter Pylori gastritis and long term use of proton pump inhibitors. Am J Surg Pathol 2006; 30:1581-1587

13 Peghini PL, Annibale B, Azzoni C, et al : Effects of chronic hypergastrinemia on human enterochromaffin-like cells: insights from patients with sporadic gastrinomas. Gastroenterology; 2002:123: 68-85

14 Modlin IM, Lye KD, Kidd M: A 50 year analysis of 562 gastric carcinoids: Small tumor or larger problem? Am J Gastroenterol 2004; 99: 23-32

15 Weisberg J, de Matos LL, do Amaral Antonio Mader AM, et al: Neuroendocrine gastric carcinoma expressing somatostatin: A highly malignant rare tumor. World J Gastroenterol 2006; 12: 3944-3947

16 Nicau GC, Toubanakis C, Nikolau P, et al: Gastrinomas associated with MEN-1 syndrome. New insights for the diagnosis and management in a series of 11 patients Hepatogastroenterology 2005; 52: 1668-1676

17 Dayal Y, Tallberg KA, Nunnemacher G, et al: Duodenal carcinoids in patients with and without neurofibromatosis: A comparative study. Am J Surg Pathol 1986; 10: 348-357

18 Bombstein-Quevedo L, Gamboa-Dominguez A: Carcinoid tumors of duodenum and ampulla of Vater: A clinicopathological, immunohistochemical, and cell kinetic comparison. Hum Pathol 2001; 32: 1252-1256

19 Makhlout HR, Burke AP, Sobin LH: Carcinoid tumors of the ampulla of Vater: A comparison with duodenal carcinoid tumors Cancer 1999; 85: 1241-1249

20 Williams GT: Endocrine tumors of the gastrointestinal tract. Selected topics Histopathology 2007; 5030-41

21 Scheithauer BW, Nora FE, Lechago J, et al: Duodenal Gangliocytic paraganglioma: Clinico-pathologic and immunocytochemical study of 11 cases. Am J Clin Pathol 1986; 2086: 559-556

22 Okubo Y, Wakayama M, Nemoto T, et al: Literature survey on epidemiology and pathology of Gangliocytic paraganglioma. BMC Cancer 2011; 11: 187

23 Burke AP, Thomas RM, Elsayed AM, Sobin LH; Carcinoids of the jejunum and ileum: An immunohistochemical and clinicopathological study of 167 cases. Cancer 1997; 79: 1086-1093

24 Soga J: Early-stage carcinoids of the gastrointestinal tract; An analysis of 1914 reported cases. Cancer 2005; 103: 1587-1595

25 Modlin IM, Champaneria MC, Chen AK, Kidd M; A three decade analysis of 3,914 small intestinal neuroendocrine tumors: The rapid pace of no progress. Am J Gastroenterol 2007; 102: 1464-1473

26 Modlin IM, Kidd M, Latich I, et al: Current status of gastrointestinal carcinoids. Gastroenterology 2005; 128: 1717-1721

27 Spread C, Berkel H, Jewel L, et al: Colon carcinoid tumors: A population based study. Dis Colon Rectum 1994; 37:482-491

28 Soga J: Carcinoids of the colon and ileo-cecal region: A statistical evaluation of 363 cases collected from the literature J Exp Clin Cancer Res 1998; 17: 139-148

29 Federspiel BH, Burke AP, Sobin LH, Shekika KM: Rectal and colonic carcinoids:A clinicopathological study of 84 cases. Cancer 1990: 65: 135-140

30 Modlin IM, Sandor A: An analysis of 8305 cases of carcinoid tumors. Cancer 1997: 79: 813-829

31 Burke M, Shepherd N, Mann CV: Carcinoid tumors of rectum and anus. Brit J Surg 1987; 74: 358-361

32 Rosenberg JM, Welch JP: Carcinoid tumors of the colon. A study of 72 patients. Am J Surg; 1985; 149: 775-779

33 Stinner B, Kisker O, Zeilke A, Rothmund M: Surgical management for carcinoid tumors of small bowel,, appendix, colon & rectum. World J Surg 1996; 20: 183-188

34 Jetmore AB, Ray JE, Gathright IB, et al: Rectal carcinoids, the most frequent carcinoid tumor. Dis Colon Rectum 1992; 35: 717-725

35 Tchana-Sato V, Detry O, Polus M, et al: Carcinoid Tumor of the Appendix: A consecutive series from 1237 appendectomies. World J Gastroenterol 2006; 12:669-96701

36 Givi B, Pommeir SJ, Thompson AK, et al: Operative resection of carcinoid neoplasms in patients with liver metastases yields significantly better survival. Surgery 2006; 140: 891-897

37 Car NJ, Sobin LH: Neuroendocrine tumors of the appendix. Semin Diagn Pathol 2004; 21: 108-119

38 Toumpanakis C, Sstandish RA, Baishnab E, et al: Goblet cell carcinoid tumors (adenocarcinoid) of the appendix. Dis Colon Rectum 2007; 50: 315-322

39 Warkel RL, Cooper PH, Helwig EB. Adenocarcinoid, a mucin-producing carcinoid tumor of the appendix: a study of 39 cases. Cancer 1978; 42:2781–2793.

40 Tang LH, Shia J, Soslow RA, et al: Pathologic classification and clinical behavior of the spectrum of goblet cell carcinoid tumors of the appendix. Am J Surg Pathol. 2008;32: 429–1443.

41 Burke AP, Sobi LH, Federspiel BH, et al: Goblet cell carcinoids and related tumors of the vermiform appendix. Am J Clin Pathol 1990; 94: 27-35

42 Griniatsos J, Michail O: Appendiceal neuroendocrine tumors: Recent insights and clinical implications. World J Gastrointest Oncol 2110; 2: 192-196

43 Larson Li. Pancreatic endocrine tumors. Hum Pathol 1978; 9:401-426

44 Kloppel G, Heitz PU. Tumors of the endocrine pancreas in Fletcher CMD Diagnostic histopathology of Tumors, 2007: Volume 2, Third edition, Churchill Livingstone

45 Heitz PU, Bordi C, Komminath P,et al. WHO classification of Tumors, Pathology and Genetics : Tumors of Endocrine Organs. Delellis PA, Lloyd RV, Heitz PU, Eng C (Eds) IARC press Lyon, 2004

46 Capella C, Heitz PU, Hopfler H, et al. Revised classification of neuroendocrine tumors of lung, pancreas and gut Virchow Arch 1995; 425:547-560

47 Deshpande V, Castilla CFD, Muzikansky, et al. Cytokeratin 19 Is a Powerful Predictor of Survival in Pancreatic Endocrine Tumors. Am J Surg Pathol 2004; 28:11145-1153

48 Tong-Hua L, Tseng HC, Zhu Yu, et al Insulinoma: An immunocytochemical and morphological analysis of 95 cases. Cancer 1985; 56:1420-1429

49 Stephanini P, Carboni M, Pathrossi N, et al. Beta islet cell tumors of the pancreas: results of a study of 1067 cases. Surgery 1974; 75:597-609

50 Service FJ, McMahon MM, Obstriet PC, et al Functioning insulinoma: incidence, recurrences and long term survival of patients, 60 year study Mayo Clin Proc 1991; 66:711-719

51 Chastain MA. The glucagonoma syndrome: a review of its features and discussion of new perspective. Am J Med Sci 2001; 321:306-320

52 Soga J, Yakuwa Y. Glucagonomas/diabetic-dermatogenic Syndrome: a statistical evaluation of 407 reported cases. J Hepatobiliary Pancreat Surg 1998; 5:312-319

53 Solcia E, Capella C, Kloppel G. Tumors of pancreas 1997, 3rd edition, Armed Forces Institute of Pathology, Washington DC

54 Fox PS, Hofmann JW, Wilson SD, et al. Surgical management of the Zollinger-Ellison Syndrome Surg Clin North Am 1974; 54:395-407

55 Deveney CW, Deveney KE, Stark D, et al. Resection of Gastrinomas. Ann Surg 1983; 198:546-553

56 Delcore r Jr, Chenung LY, Freisen SR. Outcome of lymph node involvement in patient of Zollinger-Ellison syndrome Ann Surg 1988;208:291-298

57 Stabile BE, Passaro EJ. Benign and malignant gastrinoma. Am J Surg 1985; 149:144-150

58 Gibril F, Venzon VJ, Ojeaburu JV et el. Prospective study of the natural history of in patients with MEN 1: definition of an aggressive and a nonagressive form. J Clin Endocrinol and Metab 2001; 86:5782-5293

59 Imamura M, Kanda M, Takahashi K, et al Clinicopathological characteristics of duodenal microgastrinomas. World J Surg 1992; 16:703-709

60 Sutliff VE, Doppman JL, Gibril F, et al. Growth of newly diagnosed untreated metastatic gastrinomas and predictors of growth pattern J Clin Oncol 1997; 15: 2420-2431

61 Rahier J, Guiot Y, Sempoux C. Persistent hyperinsulinimic hypoglycemic: a heterogeneous syndrome unrelated to nesidioblastosis Arch Dis Child Fetal Neonatal Ed 2000; 82:F108-F112

62 Palladino AA, Stanley CA. Nesidioblastosis No Longer! It's All About Genetics. Editorial, J Clin Endocrinol % Metab 2011; 96:617-619

63 Whittles RM, Straus IF, Sugg SL, et al. Adult onset nesidioblastosis causing hypoglycemia, an important clinical entity and continuing treatment dilemma. Arch Surg 2001; 136:646-653

Chapter 4: Tumors of Adrenal Gland

Table 4.1 Lesions of Adrenal Glands (n=387) Author's series (1970=2006)		
Tumors of Adrenal Cortex	130	
Adenoma		56
Adenocarcinoma		74
Tumors of Adrenal Medulla	202	
Neuroblastoma		75
Ganglioneuroblastoma		7
Ganglioneuroma		1
Pheochromocytoma		117
Medullary hyperplasia		2
Metastatic Tumors:	27	
Adenocarcinoma		13
Small Cell Carcinoma		6
Malignant Lymphoma (NHL)		8
Miscellaneous:	28	
Hyperplasia		11
Ectopic Adrenal gland		2
Tuberculosis		2
Cyst, simple		5
Hematoma		1
Leiomyoma		1
Myelolipoma		6
TOTAL	387	

(Cumulative data of prevalence of adrenal lesions from institutions served by the Authors: HN Hospital, Jaslok Hospital, Bombay Hospital and Surgical Pathology Centre)

Adrenalectomy

The prevalence of the lesions shown in this table is based on adrenal glands removed surgically and therefore does not reflect the true incidence of these lesions. The surgical removal of adrenal glands was carried out due to a clear clinical evidence of hyperfunction of the gland. Hyperfunction is secondary to bilateral adrenal cortical hyperplasia, adenoma or carcinoma. It is known that all three processes can occur without any excess hormonal secretions. An incontrovertible evidence of a mass lesion, particularly carcinoma, would lead to adrenalectomy. Rarely adrenalectomy is carried out for tuberculosis, and benign lesions like cysts, myelolipoma etc.

It cannot be too strongly emphasized that autopsy incidence of hyperplasia and adenomas is very high indeed and these lesions did not manifest clinically during life. Adrenal glands will be involved in generalized fungal or viral infections and disseminated malignant tumors.

Ectopic Adrenal Gland

(Synonyms: Accessory or heterotopic adrenal tissue)

A small strip of adrenal cortex can be found anywhere in the retroperitoneal region, from diaphragm to pelvis. The authors have seen adrenal rest in two cases, one near spermatic cord (Fig.4.1 A, B) and one near fallopian tube (Fig. 4.2 A, B). Celiac axis is the most common site and in some cases medullary tissue is also present (1). Other sites include capsule of the kidney and along the lines of descent of the gonads. The various ectopic sites for adrenal gland are shown in Fig. 3.

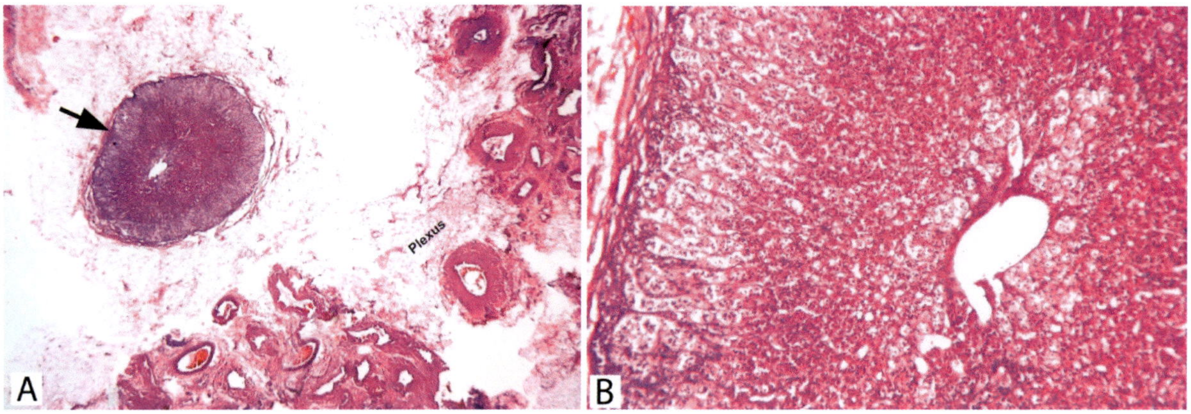

Fig. 4.1 Ectopic adrenal (arrow): (A) near venous plexus of spermatic cord; (B) only adrenal cortex is present in an ectopic gland

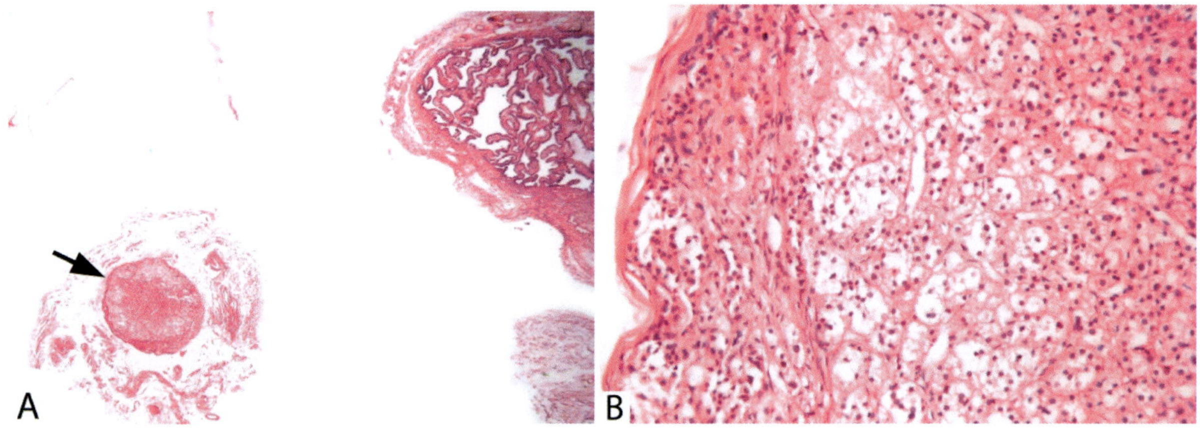

Fig. 4,2 Ectopic adrenal (arrow): (A) rest near fallopian tube (B) close up of ectopical gland: no medulla

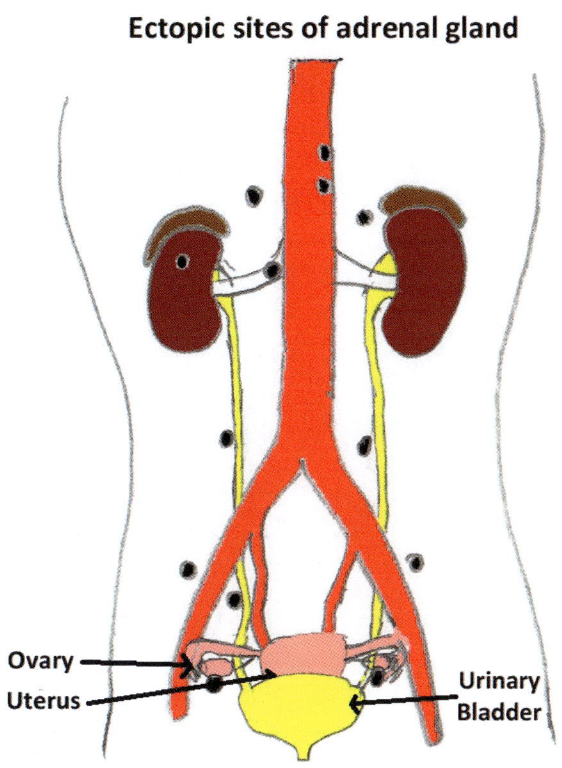

Fig 4.3 Vicinity of adrenal & gonads during embryogenesis leads to ectopic adrenals

Adrenal Cortical Hyperfunction

(Hyperplasia, adenoma and carcinoma)

Adrenocortical hyperfunction is a fascinating and complex disorder of the adrenal gland because of difficulties in clinical and morphological correlation. The process of hyperplasia is diffuse, micro nodular, macro nodular or mixed. There are problems in pathological distinction between nodular hyperplasia and adenoma and even separation of adenoma from carcinoma. Although there are numerous clinical presentations related to the adrenal cortex the morphological expressions seen by a pathologist are limited to only three, namely: hyperplasia, adenoma and carcinoma.

The clinical states in adrenal hyperfunction encountered are:

Cushing's syndrome (hyperplasia, adenoma or carcinoma)

Conn's syndrome or hyperaldosteronism (adenoma)

Virilizing syndrome (carcinoma)

Feminizing syndrome (carcinoma)

Clinically suspected nonfunctioning tumor (usually carcinoma)

Incidental findings in patients undergoing CT scan for extra-adrenal conditions

Hyperplasia

It is necessary to know the various aspects of adrenal cortical hyperplasia and its relation to cortical adenoma. The correct diagnosis of these proliferative lesions has therapeutic implications. The process of hyperplasia is bilateral and may be diffuse, nodular or nodular and diffuse.

Diffuse hyperplasia, macro nodular hyperplasia and adenoma represent a continuum of the same disease process (Fig. 4,1 A, B). The gross findings are much more informative than microscopic features. The degree of enlargement varies considerably and ranges from modest cortical thickening to large macro nodular glands weighing up to 50-60 grams !

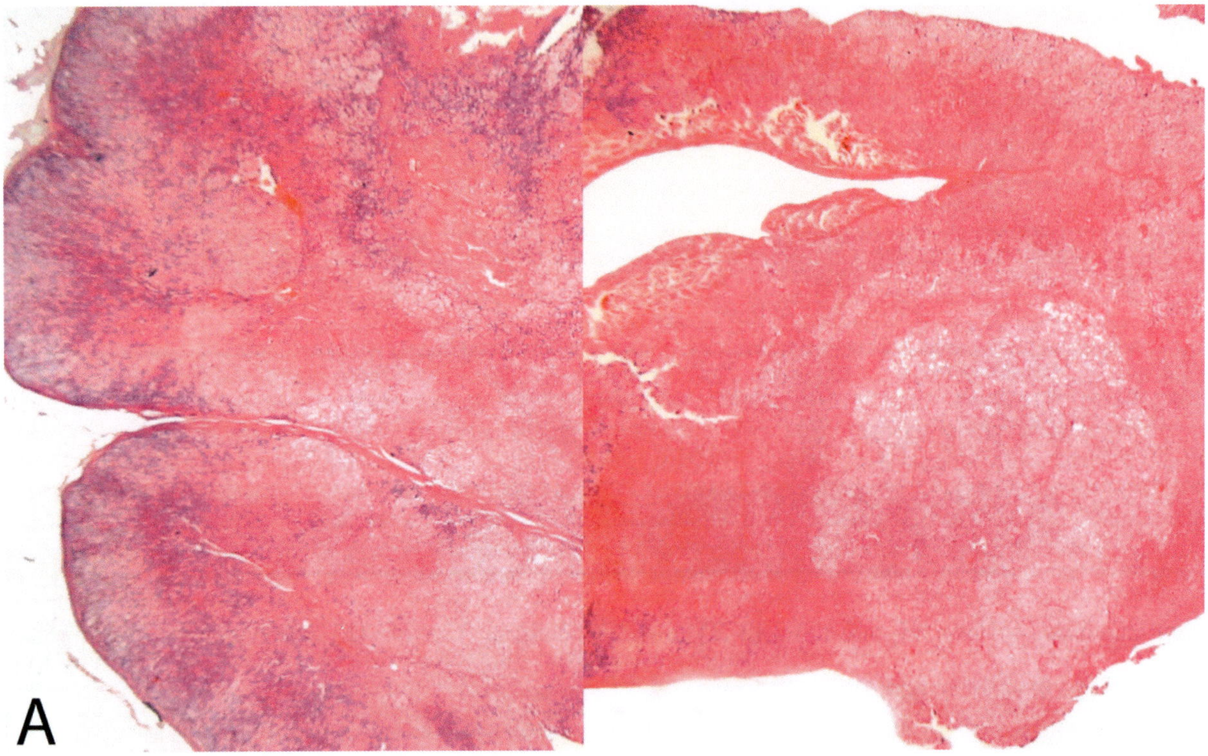

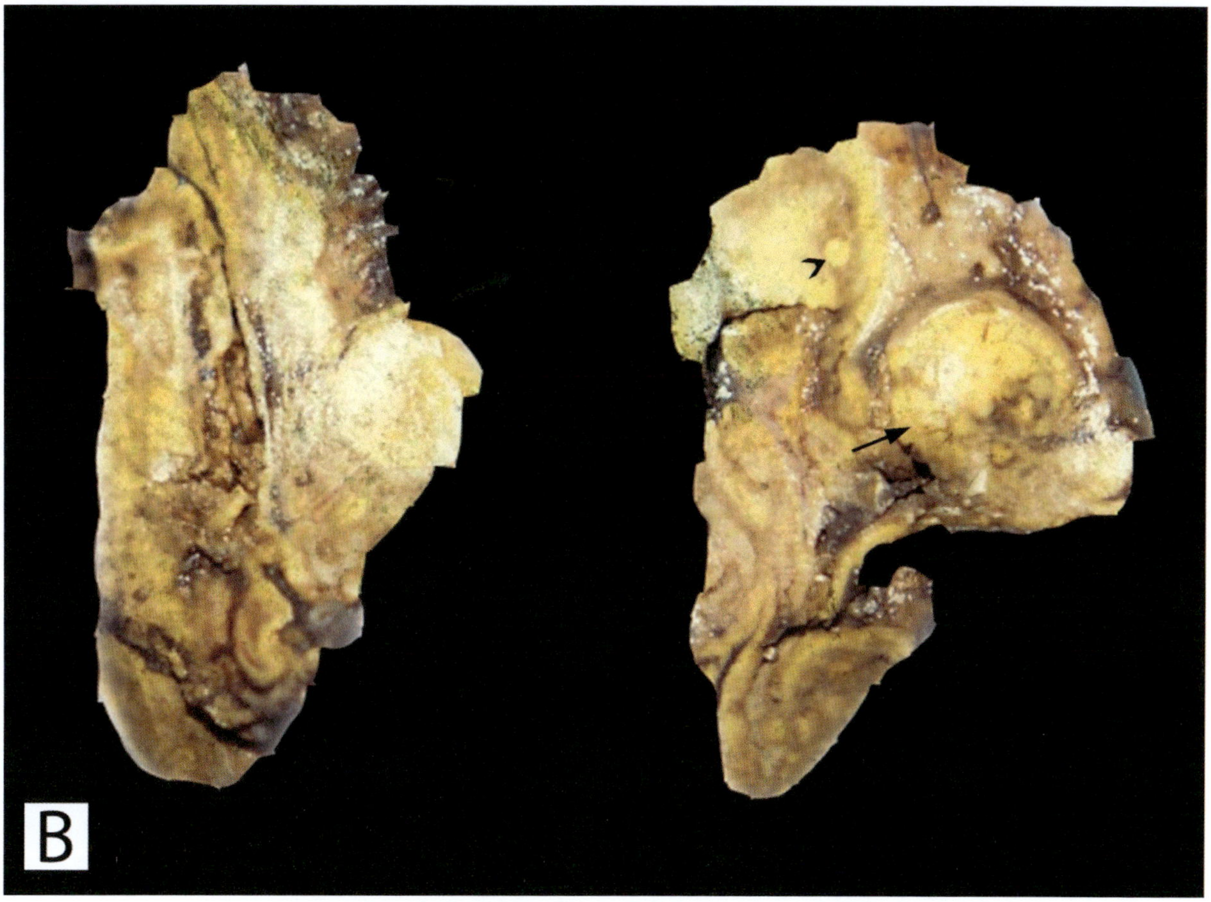

Fig 4.4 Hyperplasia of adrenal glands: (A) mixed diffuse and micro nodular hyperplasia; (B) diffuse hyperplasia with nodules, a 3 mm small nodule (arrow head) and large nodule (arrow) in a case of adrenal Cushing's syndrome

Gross:

The gland usually appears pale yellowish or yellowish brown and rarely some nodules may exhibit black pigment. In some cases, particularly on CT scan study, large nodule in a hyperplastic gland may not be distinguishable from an adenoma. However, adenoma is usually single and the surrounding uninvolved cortex is atrophic.

Adenoma:

Adenoma is usually a solitary, unilateral, and sharply circumscribed to delicately encapsulated nodule. In a large majority of cases an adenoma does not show capsule, a thin layer of adrenal cortical tissue intervening between the well circumscribed adenoma and capsule of the gland itself. It may be nonfunctioning and therefore incidentally found or associated with an endocrine syndrome. Primary hyperaldosteronism (Conn's syndrome) is most commonly associated with an adenoma, Cushing's syndrome being next in frequency. Virilizing and feminizing syndromes due an adenoma are uncommon. As in the case of hyperplasia, pathological features are not predictive of the type of endocrine hyperfunction. Basically, the role of the surgical pathologist is confined to complete documentation of the excised specimen and to rule out a carcinoma. The diagnosis of adenoma is actually established on the basis of clinical, endocrinal and radiological findings.

Gross:

Most adenomas measure from about 1.5 cm to 6 cm and weigh less than 50 g (2). Cut section shows diffuse pale yellow, golden yellow or yellowish brown tissue with larger tumors having variegated appearance due to hemorrhages and cystic degeneration (Fig.4.5).

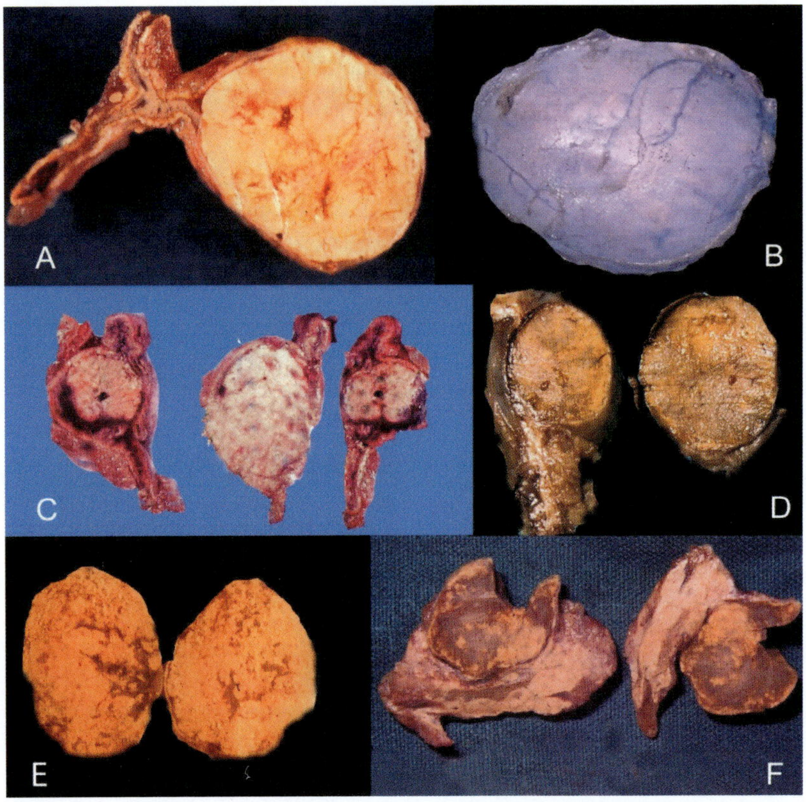

Fig 4.5 Adrenal cortical adenomas: (A) shows a classical adenoma; (B, C) large non functioning adenomas incidentally detected; (A, D, E, F) all these adenomas presented with Cushing's syndrome

Although, the gross appearance is not diagnostic of any endocrine syndrome, a few generalizations can be made. Aldosterone secreting adenomas tend to be small and measure about 1.6 to 3 cm (3, 4, 5). Adenomas of Cushing's syndrome measured 3.6 cm, on an average (3), in one series and weighed 10 to 40 g in another study (4). Occasionally adenomas weighing more than 100 g have been reported in Cushing's syndrome.

Microscopy:

Adenomas also consist of light and dark cells in varying proportions as in hyperplasia (Fig. 4.6 A) but the architecture is distinct from the surrounding cortex. The cells are arranged in solid alveolar fashion or in short cords and trabeculae supported by delicate collagen network (Fig. 4.6 B). The sharp circumscription even without any capsule sets adenoma apart from the rest of the gland. Most adenomas have a pseudo capsule formed by condensed cortical tissue and the capsule when present may be part of the capsule of the gland itself

The medullary tissue gets pushed and slightly compressed, depending upon the size of the adenoma or else the tumor projects into the periadrenal fat. The nuclei of the constituent cells are usually small and fairly uniform, although scattered enlarged nuclei or binucleation may be seen. In some adenomas the nuclear pleomorphism can be striking (Fig.4.6 C) and even mitotic activity may also be present, which makes differentiation from carcinoma indeed difficult. Capsular and/or vascular invasion and presence of metastasis are the only reliable criteria for the diagnosis of carcinoma. A detailed discussion on the vexing problem of separating adenoma from carcinoma is discussed elsewhere in this chapter. Rarely adenoma is composed of large cells rich in homogenous acidophilic cytoplasm, the oncocytic adenoma, note large bizarre nuclei (Fig. 4.6 D).

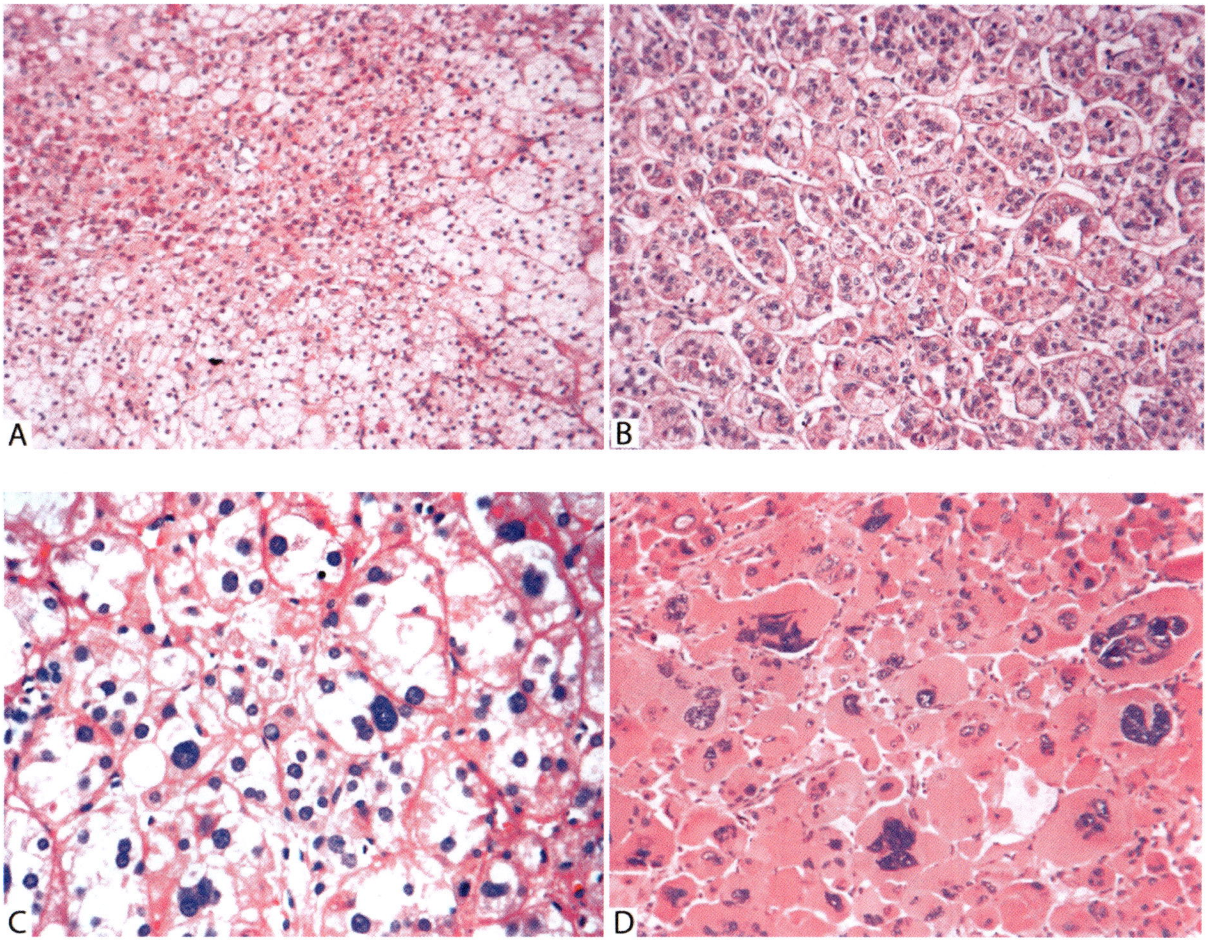

Fig 4.6 Histological patterns of adenoma: (A) mixture of dark and light cells (lipid filled); (B) cells arranged in tubular fashion; (C) moderate nuclear pleomorphism with no necrosis or mitosis; (D) oncocytic adenoma with large brightly eosinophilic cytoplasm, note bizarre giant nuclei, note absence of mitosis

Carcinoma of adrenal cortex

This is a rare malignant tumor and in the experience of large cancer registries, occurs at the rate of about 1 case per 1.7 million population or accounts for 0.02 % of all cancers (6). A large proportion of patients have endocrine syndromes and the tumor is often advanced or inoperable at the time of diagnosis. The prognosis is determined by the success of initial surgical management. As noted earlier, differentiating adenoma from carcinoma poses a challenge to the surgical pathologist.

Clinical findings

The peak incidence is between 30 to 50 years of age and the male to female ratio is slightly in favor of females. Abdominal pain, palpable mass and loss of weight are the most common manifestations. Because of the deep retroperitoneal location of the adrenal gland the tumor attains a huge size before it becomes symptomatic. Intermittent fever has been reported in 10-20% of cases (7, 8). At the time of presentation 24% to 50% of the patients may have demonstrable metastases in lung, liver or bones (9, 10). In the numerous clinical studies covering close to 350 cases of this neoplasm, functional activity has been reported to vary from 24% to 72% (8-14), Cushing's syndrome is the most frequent endocrine disturbance with associated virilizing symptoms in some, and hyperaldosteronism is the least common.

Diagnosis

A large palpable abdominal mass accompanied by endocrine hyperfunction should readily lead to a clinical diagnosis of adrenal cortical carcinoma. The non-functioning carcinomas tend to be even larger in size and will be considered as part of differential diagnosis of any retroperitoneal mass. The various radiological investigations including sonography and CT scan may be diagnostic because the tumor demonstrates evidence of invasion and even metastasis in many cases.

Fine needle aspiration cytology will be diagnostic only when florid nuclear anaplasia is expressed. However, often nuclear anaplasia of mild degree is present and is not diagnostic of carcinoma. In very advanced inoperable cases with radiological evidence of malignancy, FNAC is very useful in establishing a tissue diagnosis. FNAC has been also useful in suspected cases of metastasis in adrenal gland from a known primary.

Pathology

Gross:

Most adrenal carcinomas are of massive proportions (Fig.4.7 A, B, C,D), which are never attained by adenomas. In addition, coarse bosselations, extensive hemorrhagic necrosis and evidence of invasion into surrounding organs leave no doubt as to the malignant nature of the tumor.

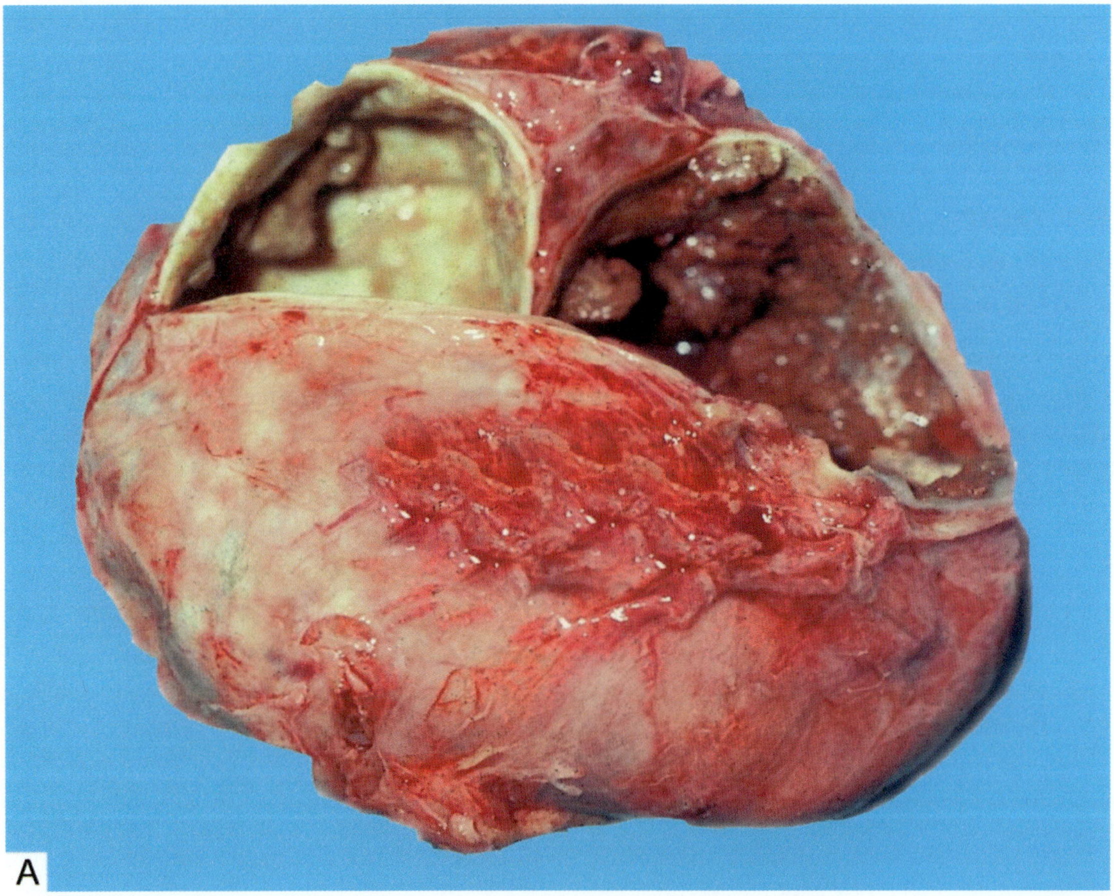

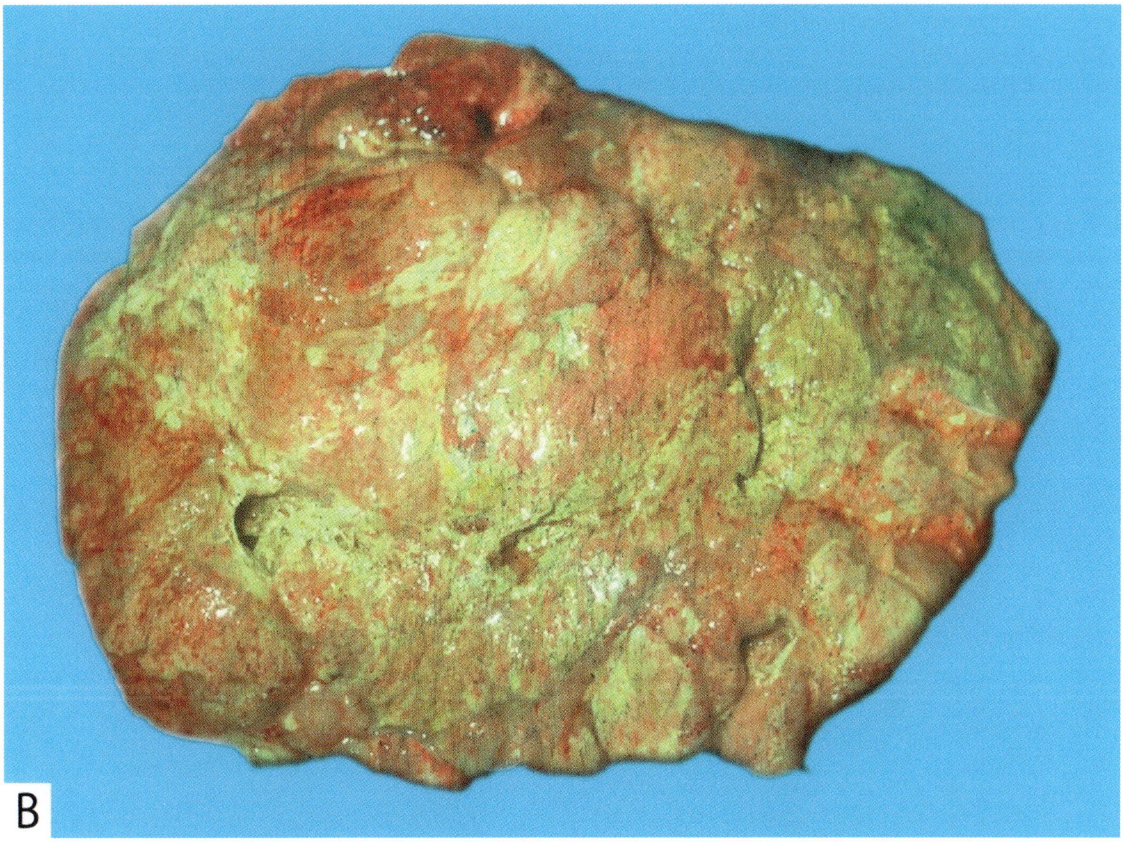

B

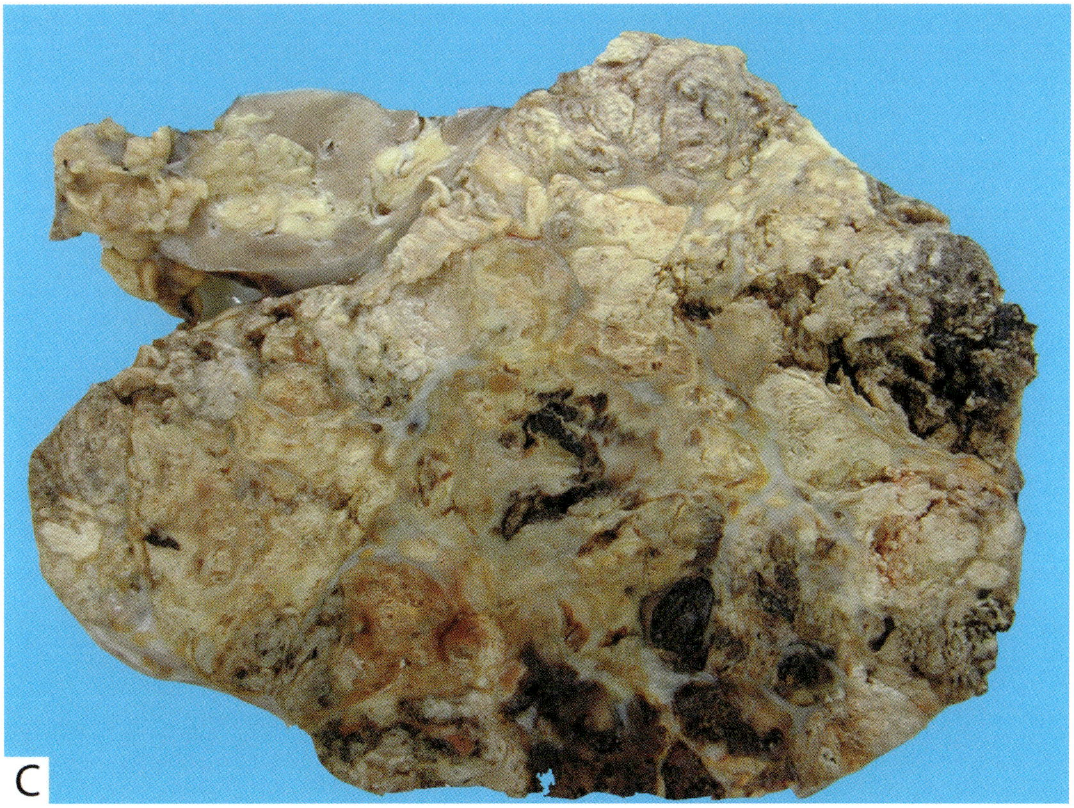

C

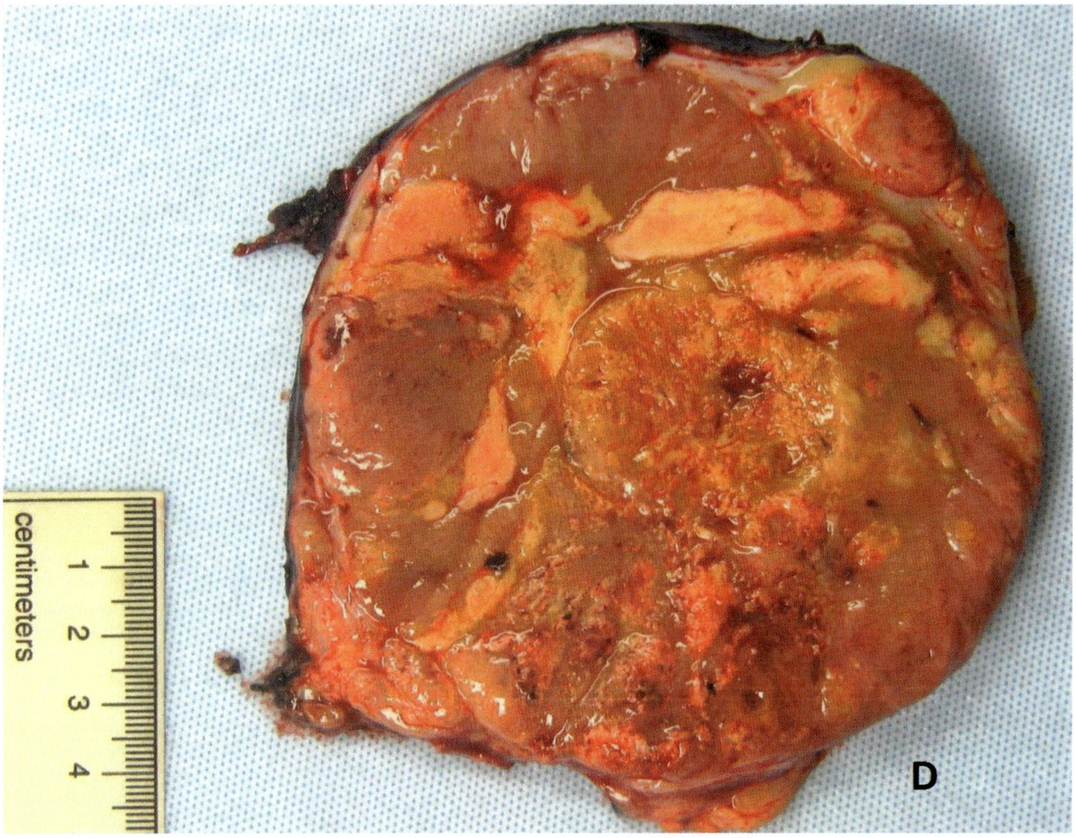

Fig 4.7 Carcinoma of adrenal gland: (A) note large size and cystic degeneration (950 g); (B) tumor weighing 560 g shows extensive necrosis; (C) 1220 g variegated tumor, note diplaced kidney at the left upper corner (D) Another example of solid adrenal cortical carcinoma, 1200 g

Sectioned surface usually shows a variegated appearance with yellow, brown and dark red colors and cystic degeneration (Fig.4.7 B, C). The average recorded weights have ranged from 100 to 3000 g in different series (9, 12, 14) According to the report of Tang and Gray, tumors weighing over 95 g were malignant and those less than 50 g benign (15). The controversy about malignancy and benigncy arises in tumors, which are well encapsulated, with no evidence of invasion and weighing around 100 g. It will be too simplistic to take weight of the tumor as an important parameter for the diagnosis of malignancy. It has been observed that the smallest tumor to metastasize weighed 40 g and the largest tumor which did not metastasize weighed 1800 g! (16, 17). Unlike in hypernephroma, only a few cases of adrenal carcinoma with invasion of inferior vena cava have been recognized preoperatively on CT (18).

Microscopic

Histological features display great diversity and the predominantly solid eosinophilic dark cell population is arranged in trabeculae, solid nests, lobules and diffuse patterns. Groups of lipid-rich light cells are present but always in a small proportion. The nuclei usually display marked pleomorphism and numerous mitotic Figures (Fig.4.8 A, B). It is important to note that majority of the cells in adrenal carcinomas are small to medium in size but reveal relatively large nuclei with high NC ratio, a very useful parameter of malignancy (Fig.4.8 C). Necrosis is often present (Fig. 4.8 D) and considered predictive of malignant behavior. The more important features in the diagnosis of adrenal carcinoma are capsular invasion, vascular tumor emboli and invasion into surrounding organs like kidney or bowel (Fig. 4.8 E, F).

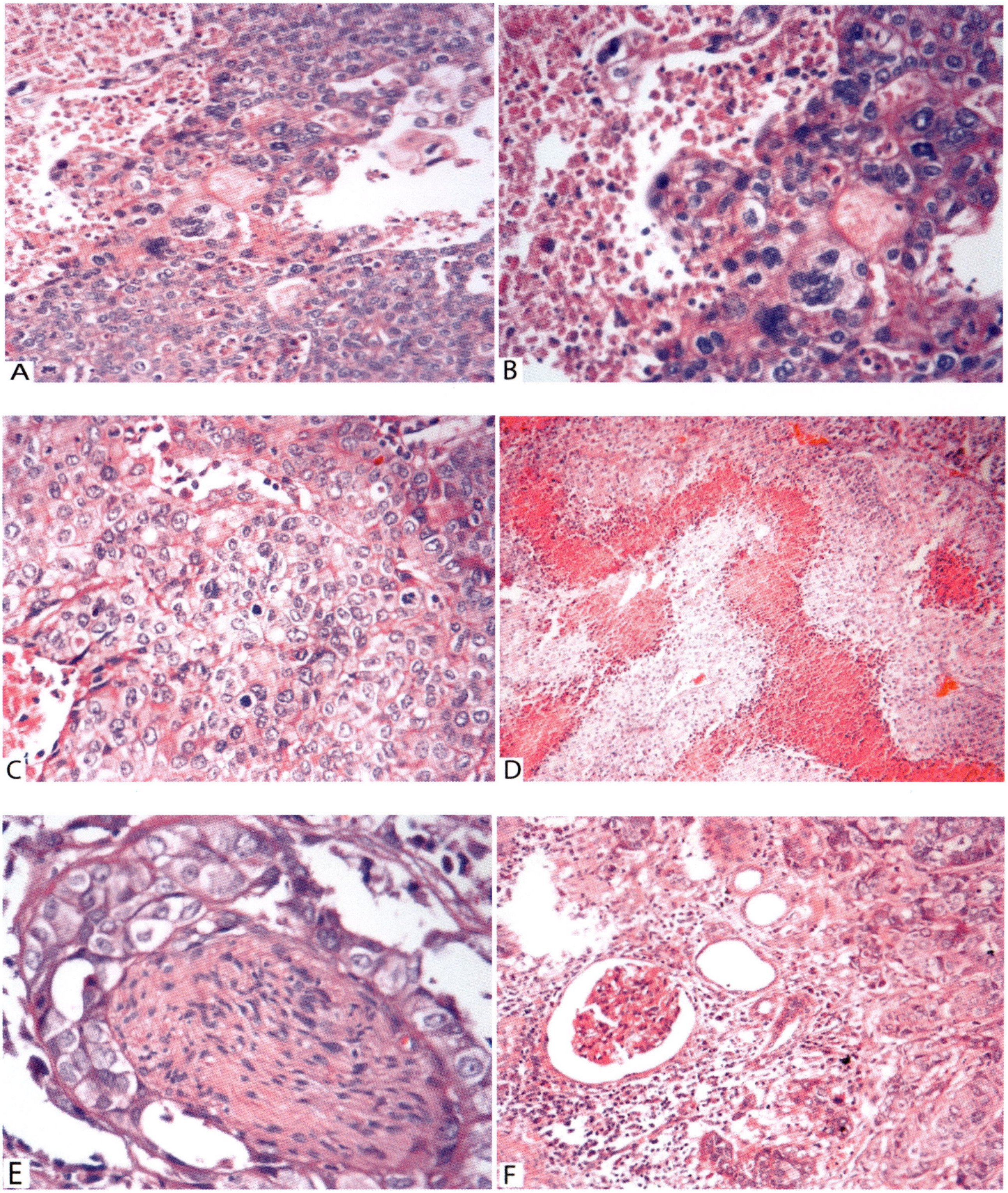
A
B
C
D
E
F

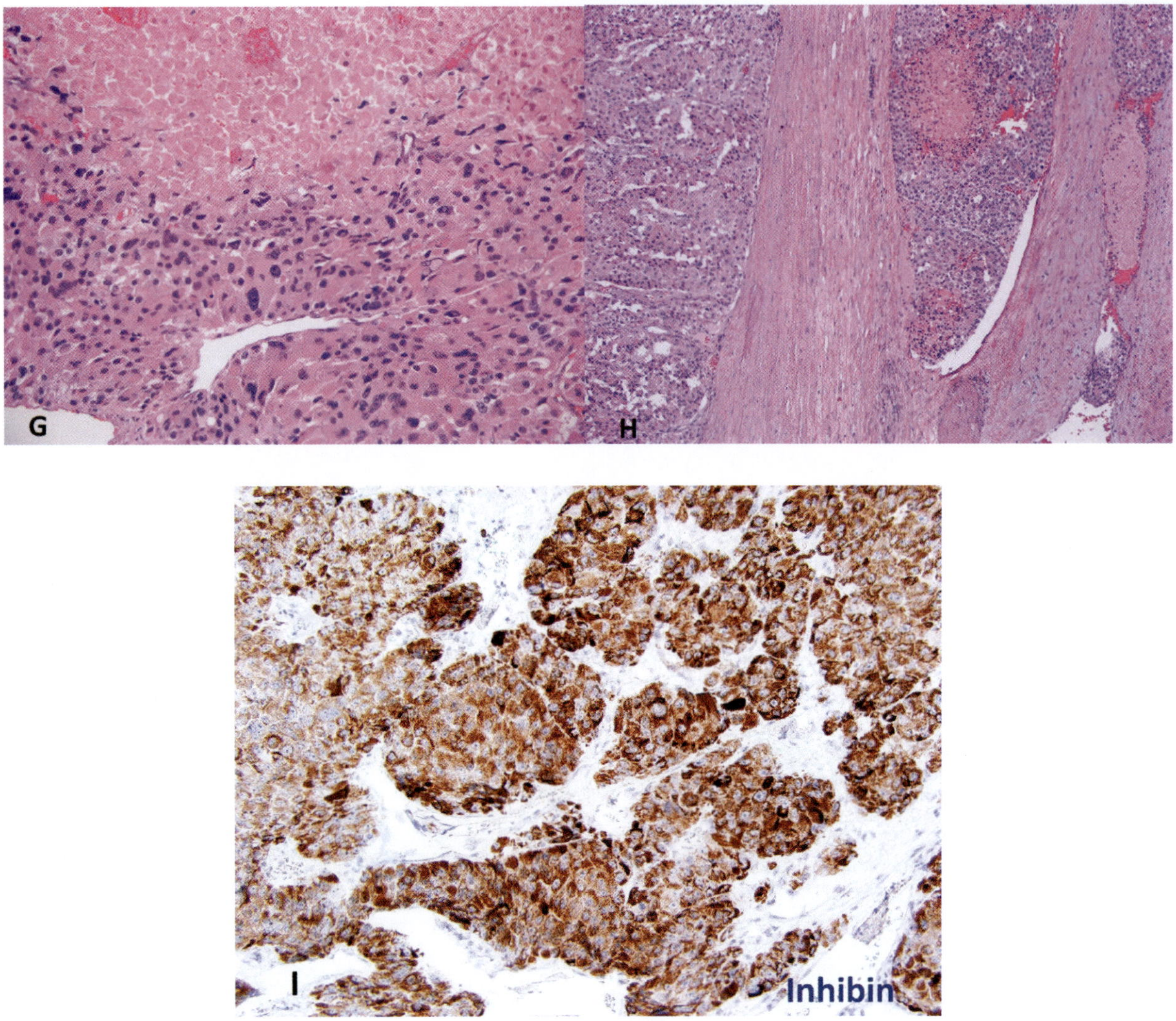

Fig 4.8 Histology of adrenocortical carcinoma ***from gross photograph A****: (A) a marked nuclear pleomorphism, necrosis and abnormal mitosis; (B) higher power of the same; (C) relatively small cells with high N/C ratio and frequent mitoses; (D) typical tumor necrosis; (E) carcinoma infiltrating beyond adrenal gland, note perineural invasion; (F) carcinoma (right half) invading the adjacent kidney. Histology of adrenocortical carcinoma* ***from gross photograph D****: (G): Focus of necrosis with nuclear pleomorphils; (H) Vascular invasion.(I) Inhibin Immnostain: strong cytoplasmic positive staining*

Adenoma versus carcinoma of adrenal cortex

Adrenal cortical tumor is one of the very few fields in surgical pathology, which requires so much effort and study to separate benign from malignant. Many investigators have devoted their energies in assessing the various criteria and defining those most predictive of malignant behaviour. (2, 12, 16, 17, 19).

Parameters of apparent decreasing importance are:

1. Presence of infiltration or metastasis found during investigations and on exploratory laparotomy
2. Vascular tumor emboli
3. Capsular invasion
4. Mitotic rate greater than 5/50 HPF or abnormal mitoses
5. Tumor weighing 100 g or more
6. Necrosis

It would appear that except for the first parameter, all other criteria are not entirely reliable indicator of malignancy and some controversial cases may have to be designated as adrenal cortical tumor of uncertain malignant potential.

Weiss, Medeiros & Vickery (20) studied in detail the pathologic features of prognostic significance in adrenal cortical carcinoma. The authors evolved a histopathological system to accurately predict the malignant potential of adrenal cortical tumors with emphasis on differentiating benign from malignant The Weiss criteria included:

nuclear grade,
mitotic rate >5/50 HPF,
abnormal mitoses,
<25% clear cells,
>1/3 diffuse architecture,
necrosis,
venous invasion,
sinusoidal invasion and
capsular invasion.

The Weiss histopathological system was applied by Aubert et al (21) to a series of 49 cases of adrenal cortical tumors and found that Weiss Score was 6.5 for malignant tumors and 1.16 for benogn tumors. Aubert modification of Weiss system consisted score of 2 for mitotic rate and proportion of clear cells and score of 1 each for abnormal mitoses, necrosis, capsular invasion. Using this system, a score of 3 or more supports carcinoma and 2 or less supports adenoma

For reasons that are not clear, tumors eliciting virilization or feminization have often been malignant (22, 23). It has also been shown by tissue culture hormonal assays that steroid precursors such as 11 deoxycortisol (S) are secreted by carcinomas but not by adenomas.

Flow cytometry: in most malignant tumors presence of DNA aneuploidy is highly suggestive of aggressive behavior. In surgically resectable carcinomas Hosaka et al (24) found that tumors with diploid DNA had more favorable clinical course than those with tetraploid DNA.

Differential diagnosis of Adrenal cortical carcinoma:

Adrenal cortical carcinoma will have to be differentiated from renal cell carcinoma and hepatocellular carcinoma (Fig. 4.9) in cases of huge tumors involving the surrounding organs. The problem will also arise when tissue from an apparent metastatic tumor is submitted for histological diagnosis. In hepatocellular carcinoma immunohistochemical stains for alpha fetoprotein, alpha 1-antitrypsin, Hep par OCH 3 and CEA will be very helpful. In renal carcinomas, cytokeratins, vimentin, CD10, RCC1 and epithelial membrane antigens can be demonstrated and these will be absent in adrenal cortical carcinoma. The latter will express vimentin, inhibin, Melan A.

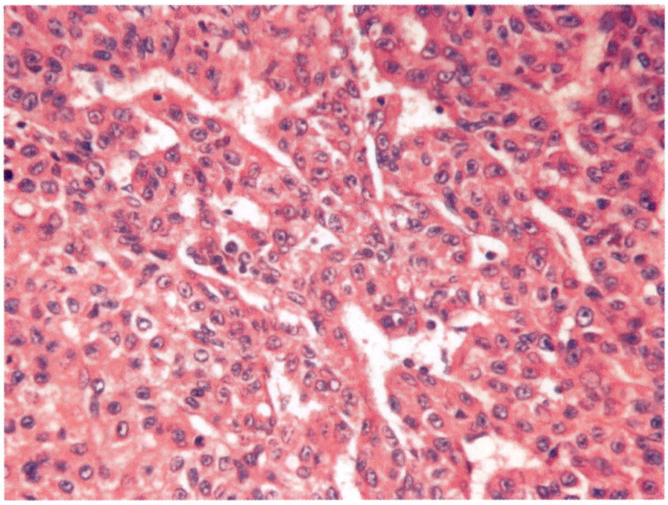

Fig 4.9 Adrenal cortical carcinoma: resembling hepatocellular carcinoma, note neoplastic hepatocytes in trabeculae separated by sinusoids

Sites of Metastasis of adrenal cortical carcinoma

Metastases have been reported frequently in liver (50%), regional lymph nodes (40%) and lung (40%). They have been also reported, albeit infrequently, in pleural and peritoneal surfaces, bones and skin particularly in anaplastic tumors. When metastasis is the presenting sign of an adrenocortical carcinoma a definitive histological diagnosis will be very difficult. In the case illustrated below the patient presented with a mass in the scapula and primary could not be identified on H & E stained biopsy slide. Immunohistochemistry (Fig. 10A, B, C, D) was diagnostic of adrenal cortical carcinoma.

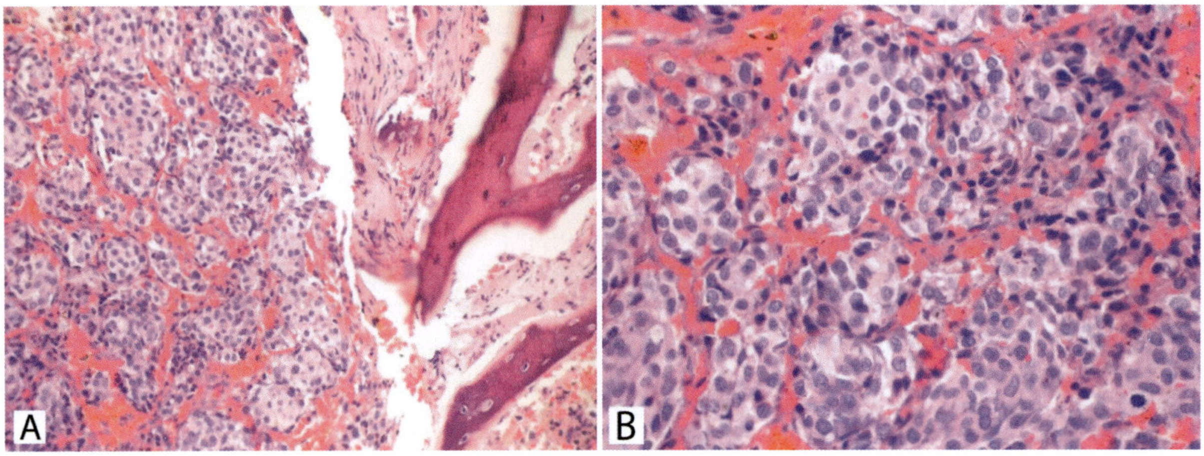

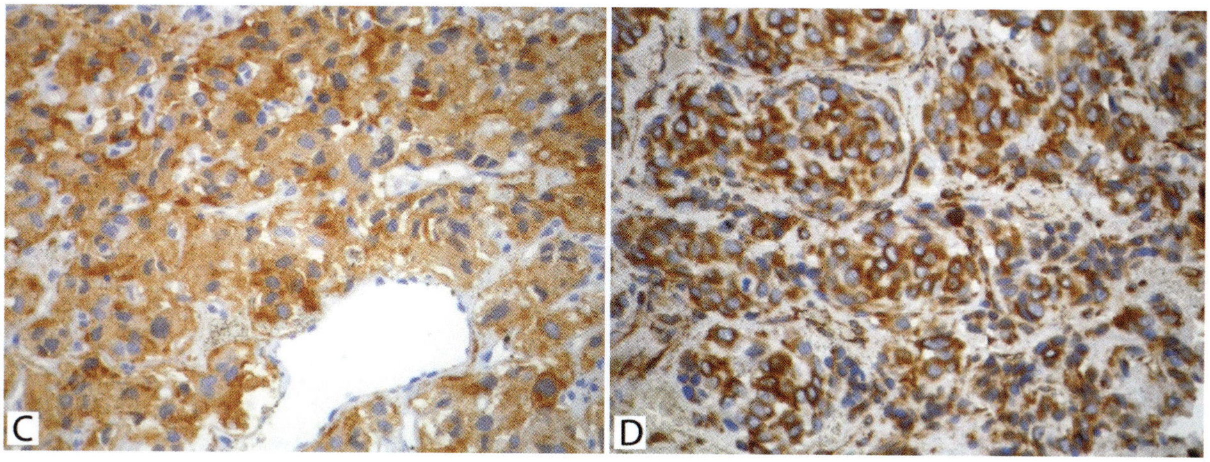

Fig 10 Metastatic adrenocortical carcinoma in scapula: (A & B) H & E morphology: differentiation from other carcinomas is not possible; (C) Inhibin is immunoreactive in cytoplasm; (D) Vimentin is strongly expressed in cytoplasm. Courtesy: Dr. Anita Borges, Raheja hospital, Mumbai, India

Staging of adrenocortical carcinoma

The staging classification used by Henley et al (8) is a modified version of the one originally used by MacFarlane (17). It compares with TNM system of staging as follows:

Table 4.2: Staging of adrenocortical carcinoma			
Stage I	T1 - Tumor 5 cm or less, no local invasion	N0	M0
	T2 - Tumor 5 cm or more, no local invasion.	N0	M0
Stage II	T3 - Tumor any size but locally invasive. Adjacent organs not involved.	N0	M0
Stage III	T4- Tumor any size invading adjacent organ	N0	M0
Stage IV	N1- Positive regional lymph nodes	N1	
	M1-Distant metastasis	M1	

Prognosis

The 5 year survival figures in adrenal carcinoma are dismal and in four large reviews 70% to 78% of the patients succumbed to the disease (9, 10, 11, 13); in another set of studies the mortality rate ranged from 81 to 88% (8, 15, 25, 26). As in any other malignant tumors survival is to some extent determined by the stage of the disease. In two series using TNM classification nearly 69% cases were found to be in stages III and IV (8,14).

Incidental nodule (adenoma) at autopsy

Non-functioning adrenal cortical nodule or adenoma (Fig.4.11) is much more frequent than those associated with hyperfunction. The incidence at autopsy varies depending upon the definition (basically size) of the nodule and the proportion of elderly population in the study. In large series with several thousand consecutive autopsies an incidence of 1.5 to 2.9% has been reported). The incidence has been much higher in autopsy studies involving elderly subjects and those suffering from diabetes and hypertension. No causal relationship has been established between these non-functioning adenomas and hypertension or diabetes, however (27, 28).

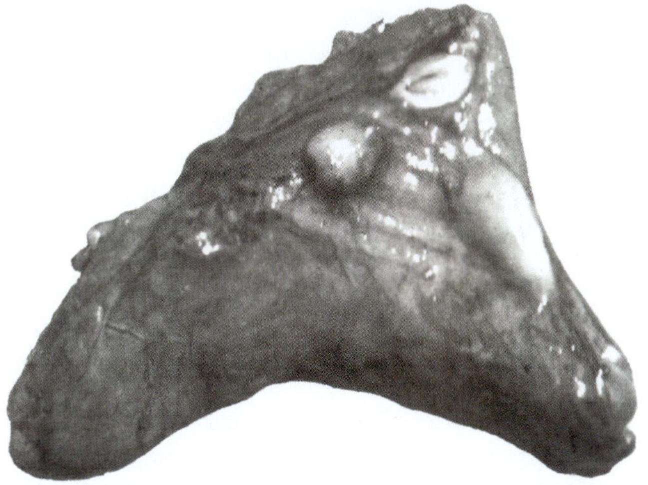

Fig 4.11 *Three nodules (adenomas) in an adrenal gland, found incidentally at autopsy*

Incidental nodule (adenoma) in living patients

With the advent of imaging techniques, as a routine method of investigation of abdominal problems, increasing number of incidental adrenal cortical lesions are being found (29). Nodules measuring from 0.5 to 1 cm are detectable on CT scan and the reported incidence of incidental nodules in large consecutive CT investigations has been 0.6 to 1.2% (30, 31). The nodules vary in size from 1.5 to 4 cm with an average of about 2.5 cm (30, 32).

In vast majority of cases, no attempt at histological diagnosis has been made. Kutz and Shikoda (33) reported 23 non-functioning adrenal nodules measuring less than 3 cm, discovered during CT examination of abdomen for extra adrenal neoplasms. In all cases fine needle aspiration cytology was carried out and diagnosis of benign adenoma was made in 7 cases and carcinoma metastatic to adrenal in 9 cases. They recommended that FNAC is to be preferred to a biopsy to unravel the nature of an incidentally found adrenal nodule

Clinical states

Cushing's syndrome (hypercorticism)

Hyperfunction of the adrenal cortex may lead to excess secretions of all steroid hormones but most commonly glucocorticoid overproduction takes place. A constellation of findings, namely truncal obesity, weakness, easy bruisability, hirsutism, hypertension, hyperglycemia, mental depression etc. constitute the Cushing's syndrome. When the syndrome is associated with pituitary adenoma the eponym Cushing's disease is employed. There are four mechanisms of causation of Cushing's syndrome (34, 35):

1. Pituitary-dependent ACTH over production (Cushing's disease)
2. Adrenal cortical adenoma and carcinoma (Adrenal Cushing's)
3. Ectopic ACTH production (Ectopic Cushing's)
4. Ectopic corticotrophin releasing factor (CRP) production

ACTH dependent Cushing's syndrome is most frequently associated with pituitary adenoma and ACTH independent Cushing's syndrome is caused by adenoma, carcinoma of macronodular hyperplasia of the adrenal gland (36).

Pituitary dependent Cushing's syndrome (Primary Cushing's syndrome)

Excess ACTH levels lead to diffuse hyperplasia or micro nodular hyperplasia of adrenal glands with consequent hypercorticism. In about 20% of cases a macro nodular hyperplasia (2) with glands weighing 15 to 60 g has been encountered. Some have large dominant nodule making preoperative differentiation between nodular hyperplasia and adenoma quite difficult. This has important therapeutic implications, since an adenoma requires excision while most cases of hyperplasia are managed conservatively.

In one series, 74% of patients with ACTH excess had a pituitary adenoma but in 17% no pituitary tumor was detected (37). Some of these cases may represent hypothalamic dysfunction in regulating pituitary ACTH production.

Adrenal Cushing's syndrome

According to Gruhn and Gould (38) 5-18% of Cushing's syndrome cases are due to adenoma (Fig.4.12 A, B, C) and 5% due to carcinoma. Associated virilizing or feminizing symptoms indicate a strong possibility of carcinoma. About 54% of adrenocortical carcinomas are functional, and of these 22% cause only Cushing's, 16.3% Cushing's with virilization and 0.7% Cushing's with aldosteronism. The presence of mixed syndromes, thus, should prompt suspicion of carcinoma rather than adenoma.

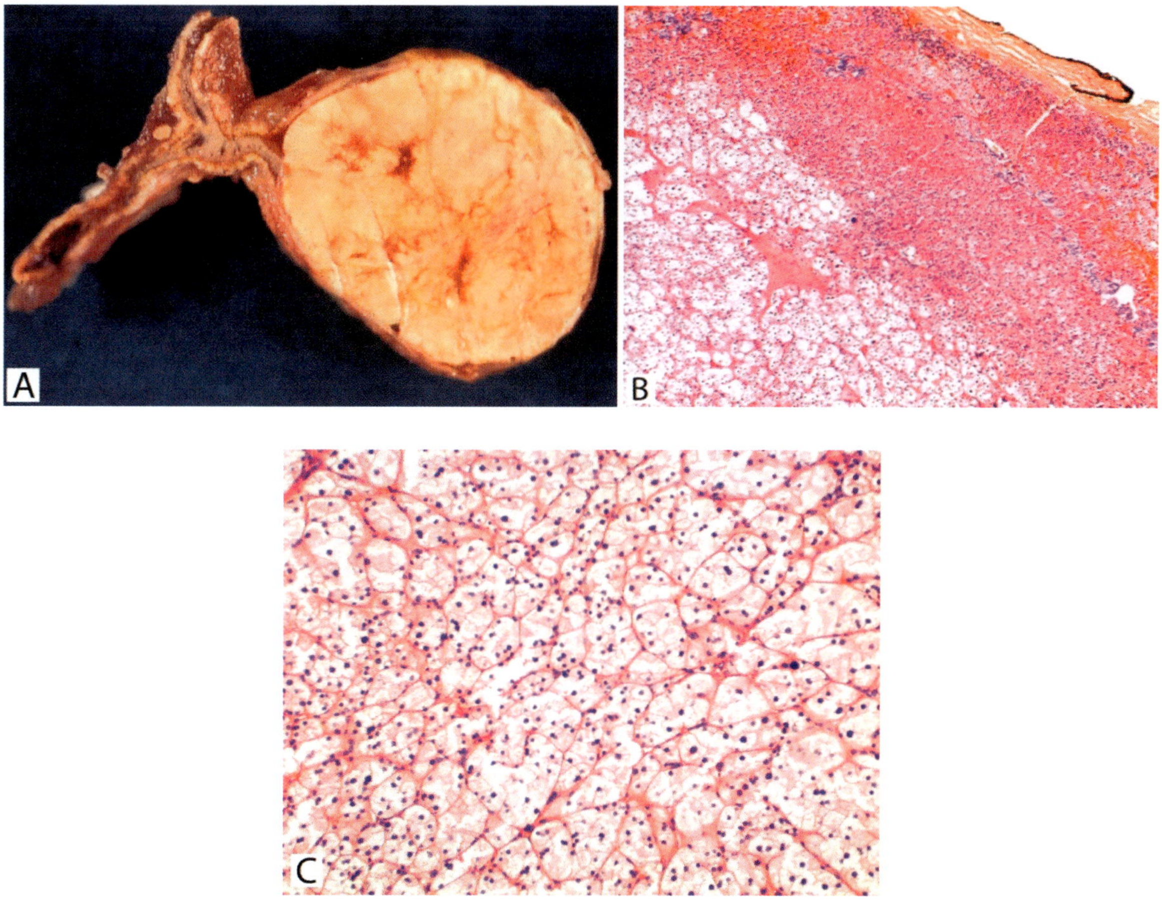

Fig 4.12 Cushing's syndrome: (A) classical gross appearance of an adrenal adenoma; (B) adenoma covered with condensed adrenal tissue with no intervening capsule; (C) large pale staining lipid filled cells in compact groups, a typical structure of an adenoma secreting hormones

Bilateral Adrenal Cushing's syndrome

90% of adrenal Cushing's cases harbour adenoma or adrenocortical carcinoma and 10% cases of primary adrenal Cushing's syndrome are associated with bilateral macronodular hyperplasia and pigmented nodular adrenocortical disease (39). The treatment involves bilateral adrenalectomy, which is curative but entails lifelong hormone replacement therapy. Alternatively, chemical adrenalectomy with drugs like ketoconazole which inhibit steroid synthesis has been successful.

Ectopic Cushing's syndrome

It is importance to know that detection of the lesion underlying ectopic ACTH production is far from easy. Ectopic Cushing's has to be differentiated from pituitary dependent Cushing's when imaging scans fail to detect a pituitary adenoma. This requires bilateral inferior petrosal sinus sampling, a test in which, ACTH level obtained from venous drainage near the pituitary is compared with peripheral blood level, before and after corticotropine hormone (CRH) stimulation. A gradient between the two locations indicates pituitary Cushing's and absence of gradient indicates ectopic Cushing's. Once this is established extensive investigations are required to detect the offending ectopic ACTH producing tumor.

Most of the neoplasms producing ectopic ACTH are clinically aggressive and often in advanced stage; undifferentiated small cell ("oat cell ") bronchogenic carcinomas accounting for about 50% cases. (38, 40, 41) In one study of 164 cases of bronchogenic carcinoma at autopsy, 10 cases, all undifferentiated small carcinomas, showed evidence of ACTH secretion (46). Jey et al reviewed their experience at Mayo Clinic and found that the syndrome was accounted for by bronchial carcinoids in 28%, oat cell carcinoma 20%, islet cell carcinoma 16%, medullary thyroid carcinoma 12%, thymic carcinoid 8%, ovarian adenocarcinoma 4%, pancreatic cystadenoma 4% and Adenocarcinoma of undetermined origin 8% (43).

Subclinical Cushing's syndrome

Subclinical Cushing's syndrome refers to autonomous glucocorticoid production by an incidentally detected adenoma with no symptoms of Cushing's syndrome. It is a topic of recent interest and controversy, because the serendipitous discovery of an adrenal mass has become a frequent event owing to routine use of CT/MRI for symptomatic abdominal lesions (44). It secretes cortisol autonomously, in a way that is no longer under control by pituitary feedback. In a cumulated series of incidentalomas, 115 patients with Subclinical Cushing's syndrome were detected among a total of 1470 cases (7.8%) (45). The clinical implications are in the form of developing phenotype insulin resistance, thus portending to atherosclerosis and its complications. Subclinical Cushing's syndrome is currently a popular term but a recent NIH conference suggested "Subclinical autonomous glucocorticoid hypersecretion" as a more appropriate designation. The controversial issue is how to treat this condition, leave it alone or remove the adrenal incidentaloma laparoscopically.

Primary aldosteronism

Conn (1955) first described this syndrome, which is characterized by hypertension, potassium depletion, alkalosis, and suppressed rennin activity. The prevalence of this disorder in unselected hypertensive population is about 1 to 2% (46). It is very important to recognize the condition, because the associated hypertension is very severe and removal of the underlying cause (adrenalectomy) is curative. Adenoma, accounting for 80 to 85% cases, typically has an orange yellow sectioned surface and a predominantly vast vacuolated cell population (Fig. 4.13 A, B). However, it is often small (Fig. 4.14 A, B) and extensive work up may be required for diagnosis. It is not possible to screen the vast population of hypertensives to detect aldosteronism. However, in patients with severe hypertension resistant to treatment and those with persistent hypopotassaemia, pertinent investigations should be carried out to confirm or rule out hyperaldosteronism.

Hyperplasia involving the zona glomerulosa is found in about 15 to 20% of cases (Fig. 4.15 A, B). An example of adrenocortical carcinoma causing aldosteronism shown in Fig.4.16 A, B : only about 20 cases have been reported in the literature (47).

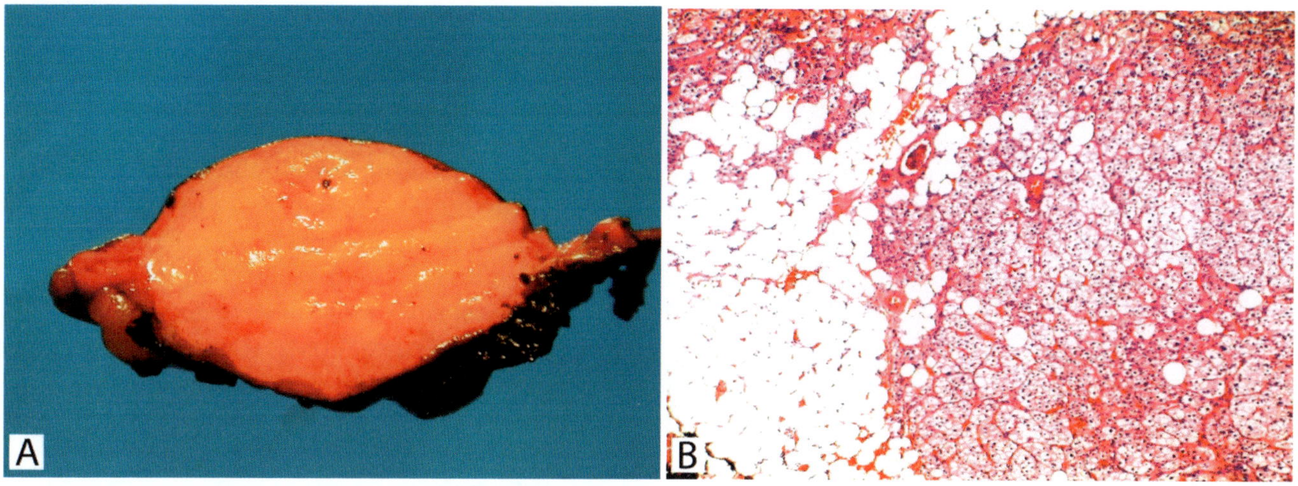

Fig 4.13 Conn's syndrome: (A) typical orange yellow adenoma (B) the adenoma has projected in periadrenal adipose tissue

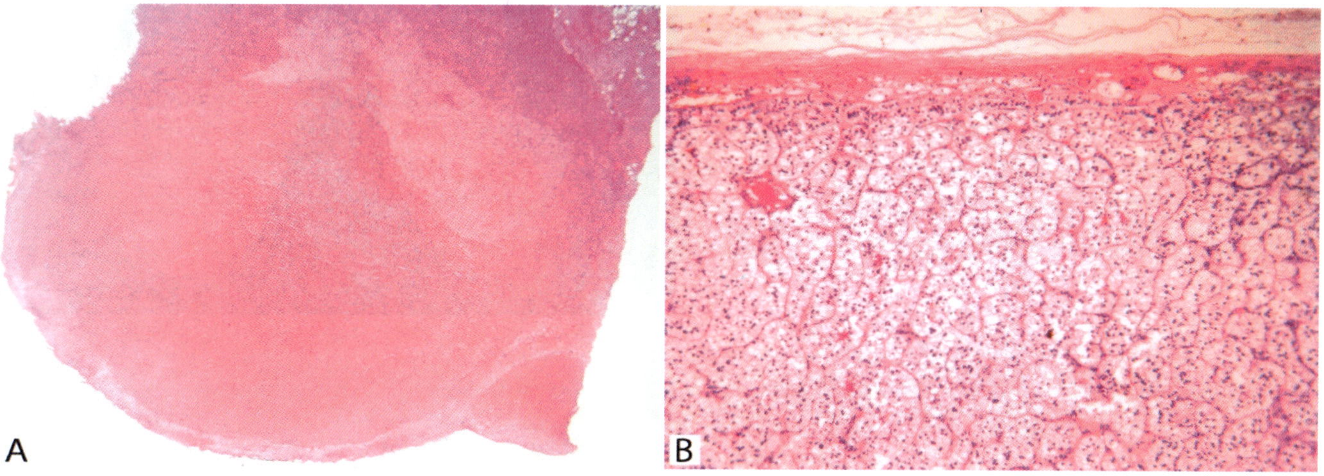

Fig 4.14 Conn's syndrome: (A) small adenoma (<1 cm); (B) a glomeruloid pattern on microscopy

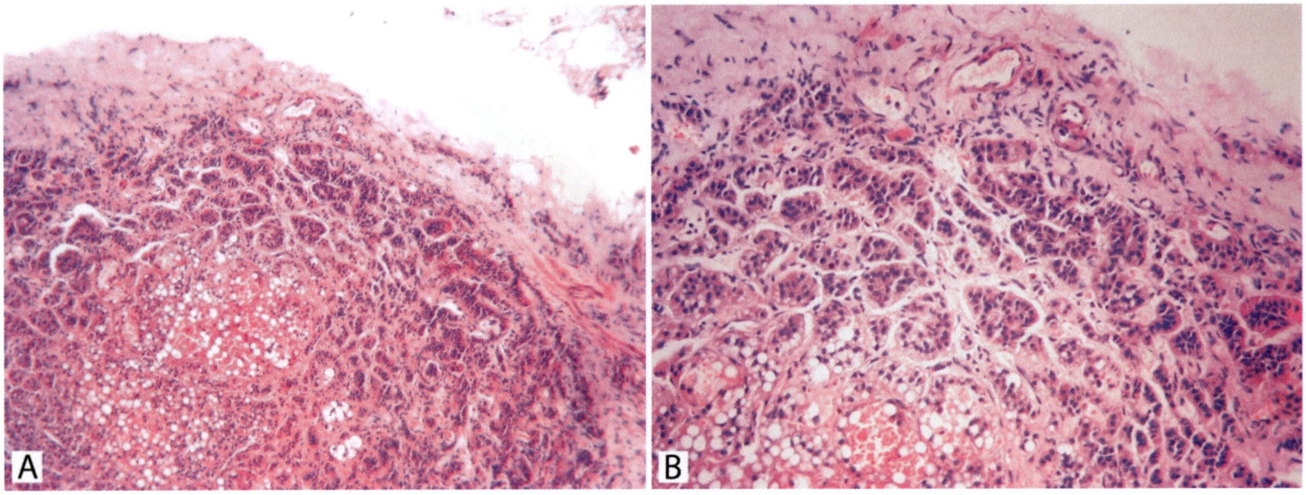

Fig 4.15 Conn's syndrome: (A, B) hyperplasia of zona glomerulosa; (normal zona glomerulosa is a very thin 1-2 layer band of constituent cells), note lipid filled cells of zona fasciculata at the base

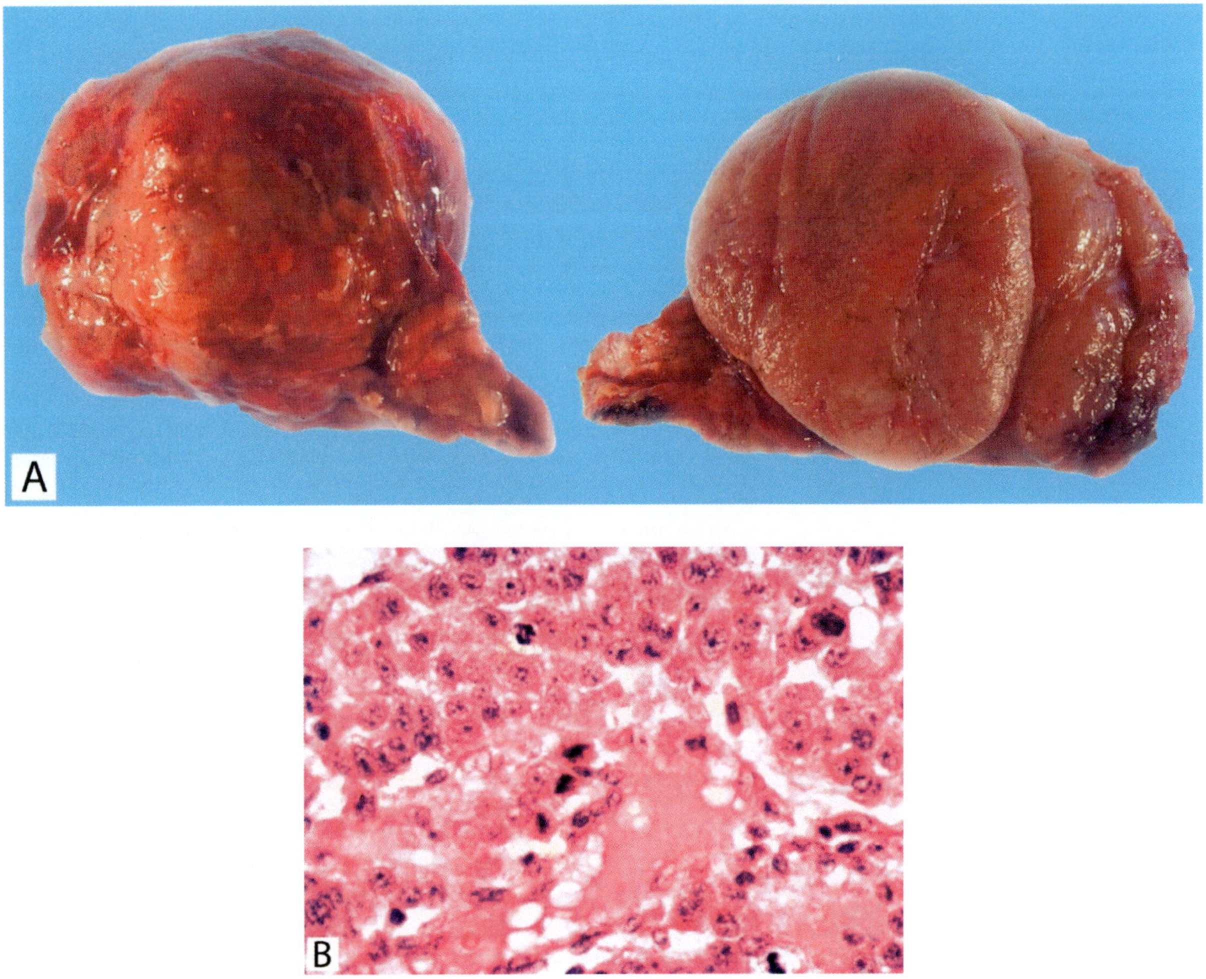

Fig 4.16 Conn's syndrome: (A) Gross: mass proved to be an adrenal cortical carcinoma; (B) Severe nuclear anaplasia with numerous mitotic figures and high N/C ratio

In patients treated with the aldosterone antagonist spironolactone, cells of the zona glomerulosa contain rounded intra-cytoplasmic inclusions. The term spironolactone body was proposed and later the inclusion was also found in an aldosteronoma. It is rich in lipids and on electron microscopy tightly packed tubules of endoplasmic reticulum are seen (48, 49).

Virilizing syndrome

Virilization refers to adult masculine characteristics occurring in a prepubertal male. In case of females, however, it will manifest at any age. Virilization in a female infant leads to severe genital abnormalities from clitoris-megaly to pseudo-hermaphroditism and is almost always associated with congenital adrenal hyperplasia. There is high level of ACTH due to reduced or lack of production of cortisol due to enzymatic deficiency leading to congenital adrenal cortical hyperplasia. Most common deficiency is of 21-hydroxylase, an enzyme that catalyzes the second last step in the synthesis of cortisol, leading to accumulation of the steroid precursors which then are used up in synthesis of androgens. This leads to marked life threatening deficiency of glucocorticoids and even mineralocorticoids occurs in addition o virlizing syndrome.

Virilizing tumors occur in both pediatric and adult age group with nearly equal frequency. Majority of Virilizing adrenal tumors in adults are malignant (Fig.4.17 A, B, C).

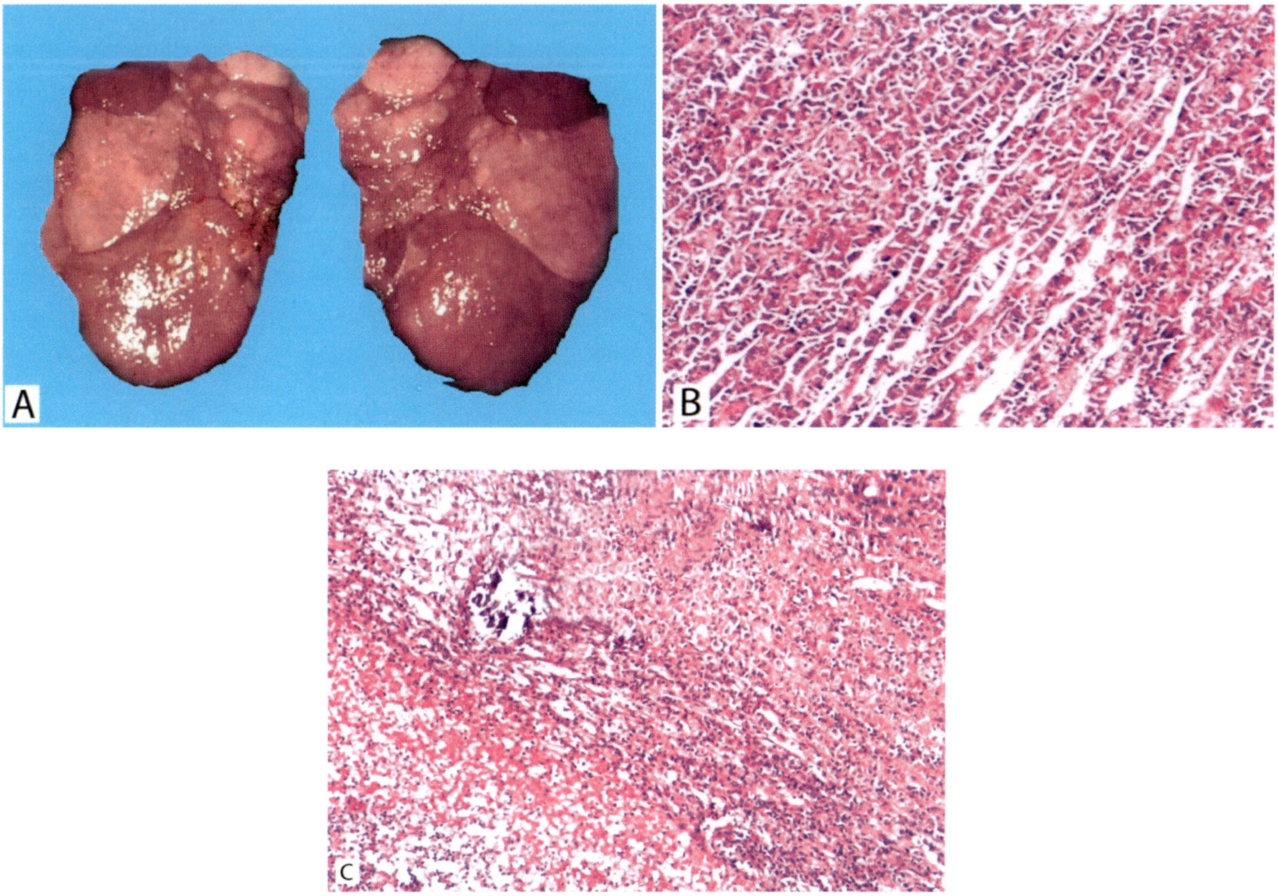

Fig 4.17 Virilizing tumor of adrenal: (A) nodular soft reddish fleshy tumor with an area of hemorrhagic necrosis; (B) tumor cells devoid of fat and arranged in cord pattern; nuclear hyperchromatism and N/C ratio are high; (C) zone of tumor necrosis in left lower corner and a focus of calcification (upper left)

Feminizing syndrome

This is rarer than the Virilizing syndrome and typically occurs in adults 25 to 45 years old (50). Gynecomastia is most common manifestation and is associated with loss of libido, testicular atrophy and feminizing hair changes. Most reported feminizing adrenal cortical tumors have been carcinomas (Fig.4.18 A, B).

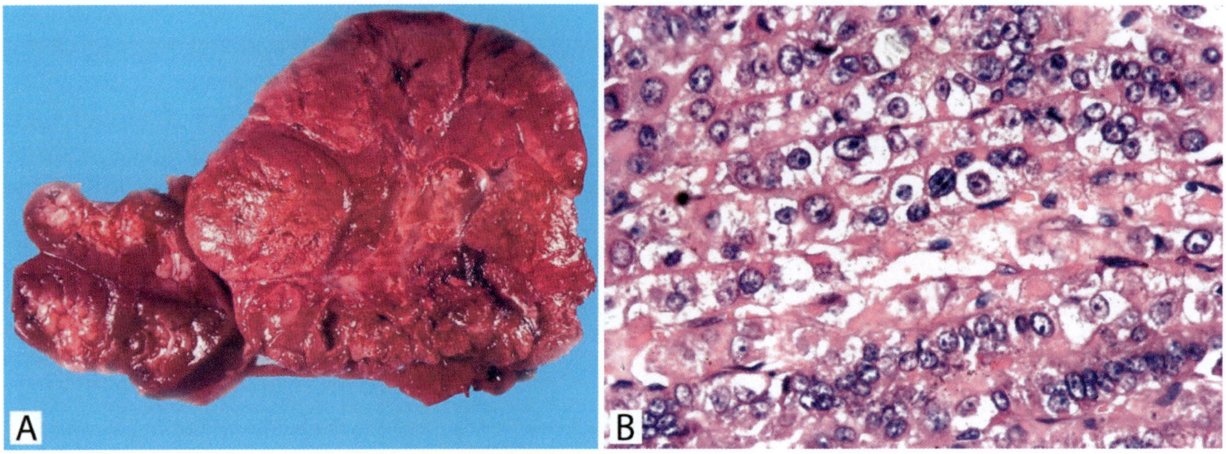

Fig 4.18 Feminizing adrenal cortical carcinoma: (A) large nodular friable tumor, weighing 875g; (B) Cells contain huge nuclei & prominent nucleoli, note high N/C ratio

Black adenoma of adrenal cortex

Small nodules or even functioning adenomas with jet black color due to presence of pigments like lipofuscin and neuromelanin have been described. The authors have seen only one example of a black nodule in an adrenal and the patient had Cushing's syndrome (Fig 4.19 A). Robinson et al (51) have reported tiny black nodules as incidental finding in 37 out of 100 cases at autopsy in adrenals of normal size. Cases of primary pigmented nodular adrenocortical disease and functioning 'black adenoma' associated with Cushing's syndrome have been described (2, 49). The presence of this peculiar light brown pigmentation (Fig. 4.19 B) has no clinical relevance. Kameyama and Takami studied the pigmented granules of black adrenal adenoma by histochemistry and electron microscopy (56). PAS with and without diastase revealed purple granules (Fig. 4.19 C) and Fontana Masson stained the granules jet black (Fig. 4.19 D). The lipofuscin pigment is the terminal product of lipid metabolism resulting from extremely active steroid synthesis and accumulates in the tissues.

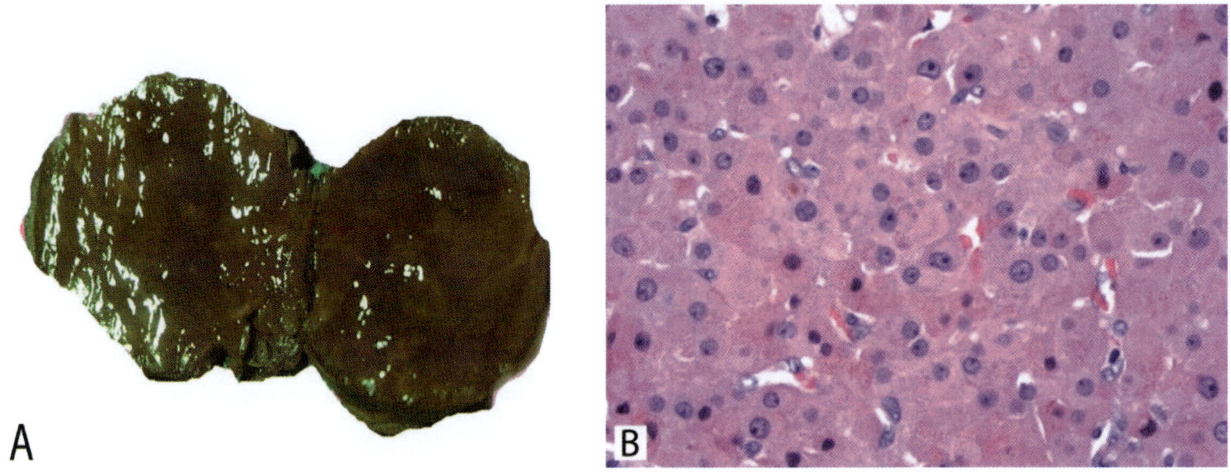

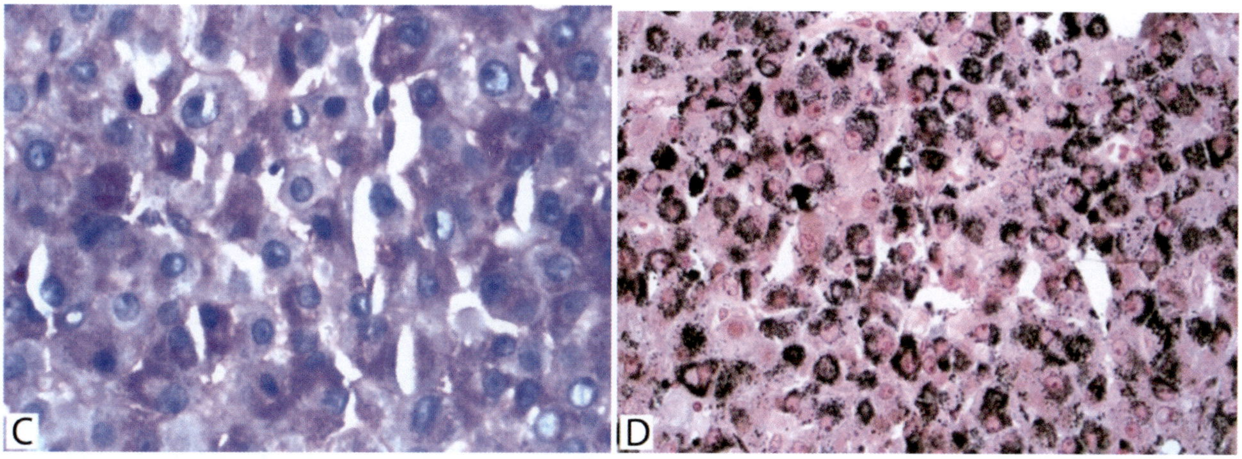

Fig 4.19 Black adenoma in a case of Cushing's disease: (A) gross picture; (B) light brown pigment in some cells (H&E); (C) faint staining purple cytoplasmic granules (PAS) (D) cytoplasmic granules stained jet black (Fontana-Masson)

Adrenocortical Tumors in Children

Some reference to this topic is germane to the discussion on adrenal cortical tumors because they are indeed rare in pediatric group and present features distinct from those in adults. An analysis of clinical features and treatment outcome of 42 cases of adrenal cortical carcinoma over a 22 year period in one center found median age of 3.9 years, a predominance of girls, virilizing signs in 90% patients and long term survival of about 50%.(53) Most reports on these tumors are based on few cases and no single pediatric center has acquired adequate experience. Liou and Kay (54) reviewed the literature and tabulated the data on 412 cumulated cases from 21 publications and the findings are as follows: median age was 4.1 years, male to female ratio 1:2.29 in favor of females, 94.5% were functional, 21.4% had metastasis at presentation and overall survival was 63.5%. The International Pediatric Adrenocortical Tumor Registry (2004) presented their data on clinical and outcome characteristics of children with adrenocortical tumors (54A). Out of 254 cases registered, 90% or 228 cases were carcinomas and only 26 cases were adenomas. The age range was 3-13 years with median age of 3.2 years The F:M ratio was 1.6:1 but it varied widely across the age groups. Approximately 90% of children had clinical evidence of an endocrine syndrome. The clinical presentations were as follows:

Table 4.3 Clinical Presentation of Adrenocortical Tumors in Children

Symptoms and signs	No of Cases (%)
Virilization	140 (55.1%)
Cushing's Syndrome	14 (5.5 %)
Mixed **	74 (29.2%)
Nonfunctional tumors	26 (10.2%)

*** includes 2 cases of aldosterone secretion and 10 cases with aldosterone + other hormones*

Modified and adapted from (Ref 54A) Michalkiewicz E, Sandrini R, Figueiredo B, et al. Clinical and outcome characteristic of children with adrenocortical tumors: A report from the International Pediatric Tumor Registry. J Clin Oncol 2004; 22:838-845

Since both adenomas and carcinoma are often hormonally active in children, making accurate preoperative diagnosis is difficult. Carcinomas are more often congenital in presentation than are adenomas and a rare one may undergo spontaneous regression (55). Distinction of an adenoma from a carcinoma without obvious metastasis is difficult in some instances, as in case of adults

Cysts of Adrenal Glands

Cysts involving adrenal are rare, usually asymptomatic, and found incidentally at autopsy. If cystic neoplasms and parasitic cysts are excluded, most cysts have no specific lining tissue and are called pseudo cysts (Fig. 4.20A, B). A rare epithelial lined cyst (true cyst) has been reported among about 300 cases described in the literature.(56) Medeiros et al reviewed 8 cases of surgically excised adrenal cysts, which measured 1.8 to 10 cm (average 6.25 cm) and had a thin fibrous wall without any lining cells. Some presented with palpable mass and flank pain (57).

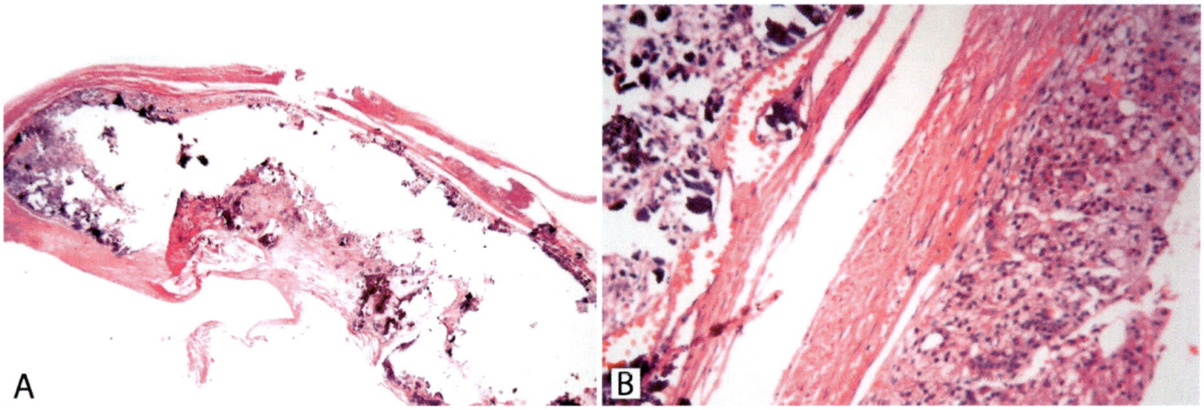

Fig 4.20 Adrenal cyst: (A) 6 cm cyst with no epithelial lining, note fibrous calcified wall; (B) adrenal cortex outside the cyst wall

Myelolipoma

This is a rare hamartomatous tumefactive lesion of the adrenal gland and consists of mature adipose cells and normal hemopoietic tissue in variable proportion (Fig. 4.21 A, B, C, D)

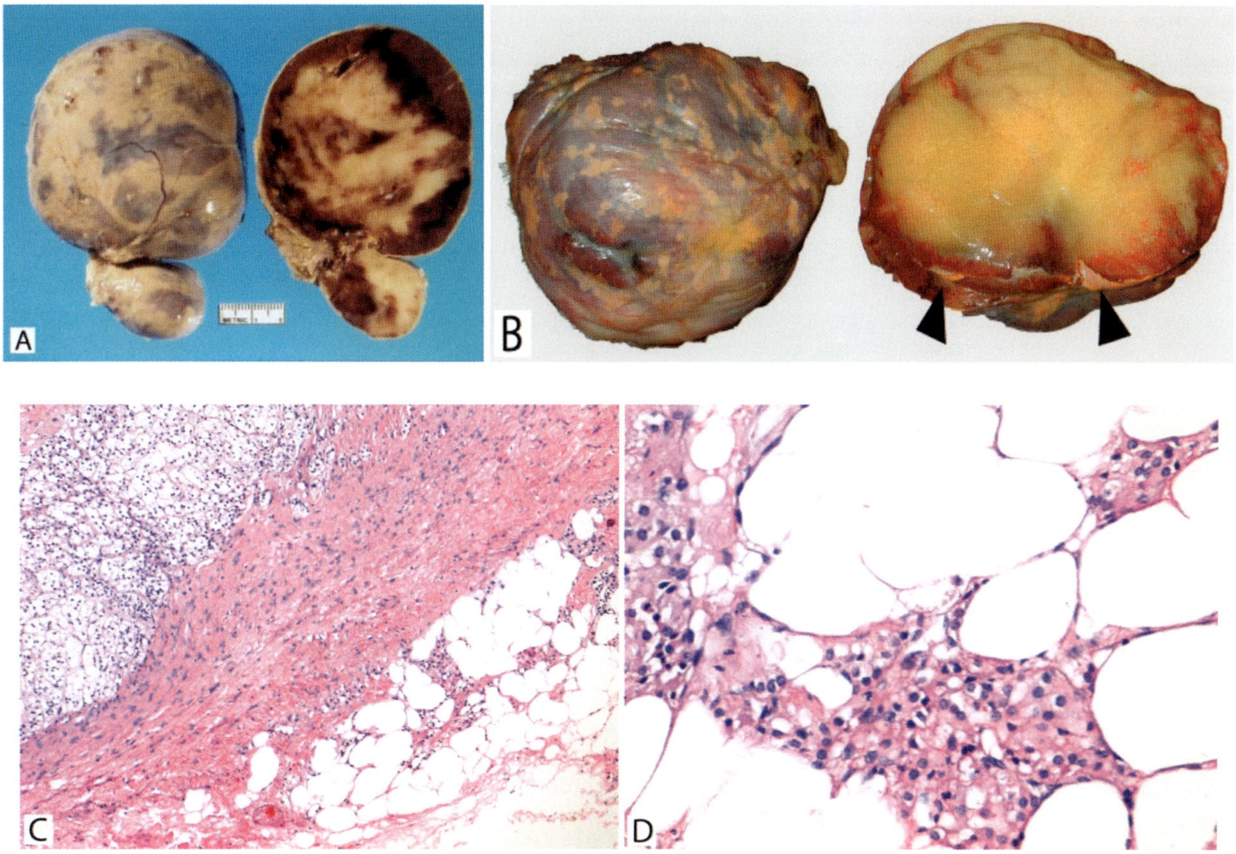

Fig 4.21 Myelolipoma of adrenal: (A) large encapsulated yellowish tumor with reddish mottling; (B) adrenal gland as a thin leafy strip (arrowhead) at the lower border of the sectioned mass, lipomatous component prominent; (C) myelolipoma has thick capsule with adrenal gland in contact; (D) hemopoietic component

It occurs as an incident finding. In one large autopsy series, the incidence was reported to be 0.08 to 0.2 % (58). In the recent years, many examples of this lesion have been found in surgically excised adrenal glands and in one series (59) half were symptomatic. These presented with flank pain in 42%, hematuria in 10%, and palpable mass in 8%. Other rare symptoms included hypertension, dysuria, hormonal disorder, retroperitoneal hemorrhage, etc. Myelolipomatous areas are often associated with hyperplasia of adenoma with a variety of endocrinal syndromes. CT appearance is the most useful diagnostic investigation. They are commonly seen in obese middle aged persons and in a study review each case was identified by inferior renal displacement on IVP.(60) In one reported case the tumor weighed 5900 g and was associated with 21-hydroxylase deficiency (61).

Neoplasms of adrenal medulla

There are no non-neoplastic lesions of the medullary tissue except a rare hyperplasia and no clinical syndrome of medullary hypofunction occurs. The adrenal medulla along with the entire sympathetic chain is derived from the neural crest. In the following schema, the histogenetic relationship of the tumors of adrenal medulla is clarified.

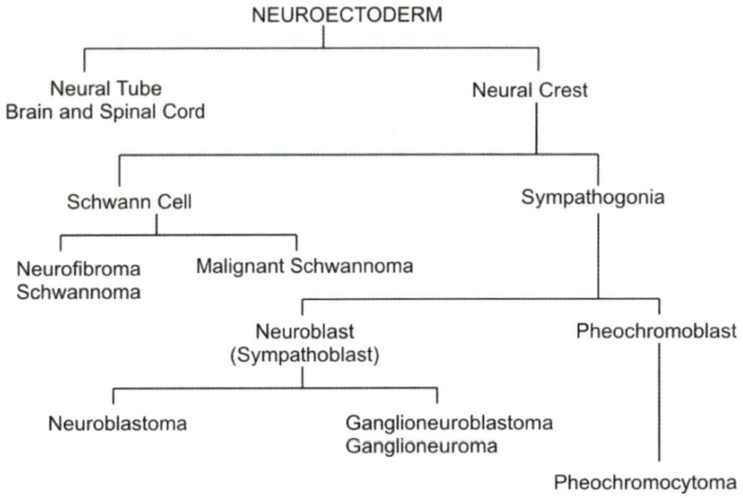

Neuroblastoma

This is the most common malignant tumor in children under 2 years of age, second only to CNS malignancies in frequency. It presents unusual biological behavior in the form of complete spontaneous regression in neonates and young children and ruthless aggression with fatal outcome in older children despite intensive multimodal therapy. It arises most frequently in the adrenal gland followed by other sites in the sympathetic system; abdominal, thoracic and cervical in that order.

Neuroblastoma occurring above age of 5 years, usually adolescents and adults, are biologically more aggressive. And they have more peripheral distribution in soft tissues and bones in addition to occurrence in the sympathetic system. However, most of those occurring in bones and soft tissues have been shown to have different molecular signature and are termed as primitive neuroectodermal tumors (PNET).

In situ neuroblastoma

Beckwith and Perrin reported a distinct tumor histologically identically to a typical neuroblastoma, which was restricted to medullary tissue of an otherwise normal sized adrenal gland (Fig 4. 22) In a meticulous study of adrenal gland, 4 examples of in situ neuroblastoma were found in 155 consecutive autopsies (62). Such a high incidence, several times the occurrence of clinical neuroblastomas, indicates that most in situ neuroblastomas undergo spontaneous regression. According to some, these nodules represent normal variation in the developmental anatomy and do not necessarily constitute an 'in situ' malignancy (63).

Familial Inheritance of neuroblastoma has been reported, suggesting a possible autosomal dominant pattern (64). Neuroblastoma has been associated with Von Recklinghausen disease (65). Maternal use of diphenyl hydantoin and excess alcohol has been implicated in the genesis of neuroblastoma and related tumors (66, 67).

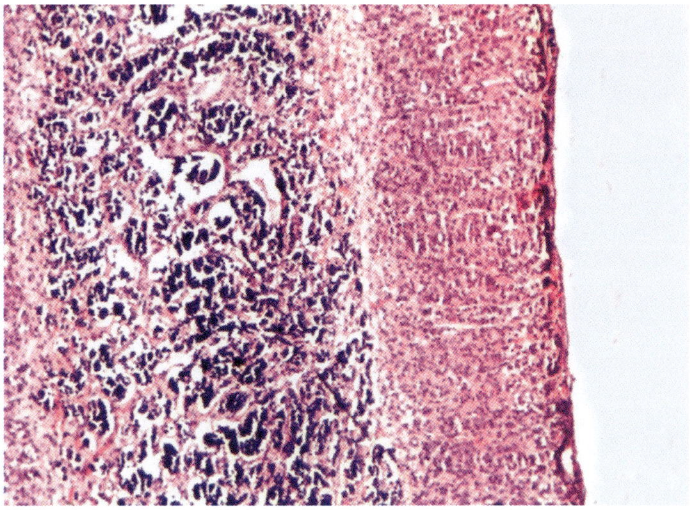

Fig 4.22 Incidental small focus of neuroblastoma: found at autopsy in case of fatal COPD, note the normal size of the adrenal. Courtesy Professor B Kandalkar, G S Medical College, Mumbai

Clinical Findings

The anatomical distribution of childhood neuroblastomas in a series of 118 cases is as follows: adrenal 38.1%, non-adrenal abdominal 29.7%, thoracic 20.3%, cervical 3.4 % and unknown 5.1% (68). The extra-adrenal neuroblastomas arise from the sympathetic chain.

Abdominal mass is the most frequent manifestation and over 60% of children reveal metastatic disease at diagnosis. Fever, anorexia, bone pains etc. are common symptoms. Infant with widespread subcutaneous grey blue nodules of metastatic neuroblastoma has been described as "blue berry muffin" baby (Fig. 4.23). Few children present with anemia and thrombocytopenia due to diffuse marrow involvement by the tumor, which is often mistaken for acute lymphoblastic leukemia. Marked hepatomegaly is found in advanced cases.

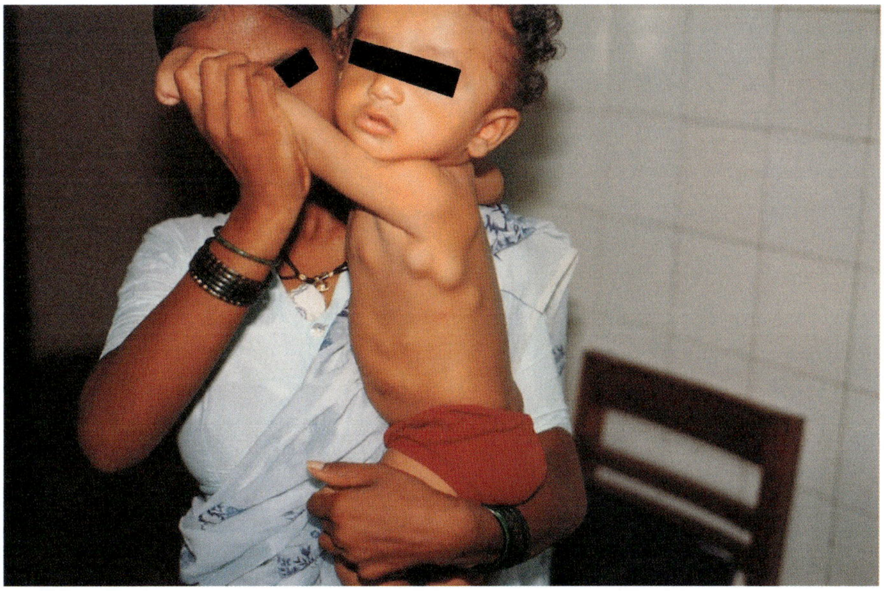

Fig 4.23 Metastatic nodules of neuroblastoma: in skin in this case of neuroblastoma, the child does not appear sick (Courtesy Dr Anuradha Murthy, Pathologist, B J Wadia children hospital, Mumbai)

Paraneoplastic syndromes like hypertension not due to excess catecholamines, severe watery diarrhoea due to secretion of vasoactive intestinal polypeptide (VIP) and acute cerebellar encephalopathy have been reported in association with neuroblastoma (69, 70, 71).

Diagnosis

VMA (vanillil mandelic acid) is a metabolic product of nor epinephrine excreted in urine and is elevated in blood in 75% of cases. Similarly, DOPA and its metabolic product HVA (homovanillic acid) is elevated in 80% cases of neuroblastoma (72). A rapid spot test for VMA in urine has been advocated as a useful test for screening of infants for early detection of neuroblastoma (73).

Bone marrow involvement (Fig 4. 24), according to one survey is found in 26% to 58% of newly diagnosed cases; some have advocated bone marrow aspirations from multiple sites (74, 75). This appears logical, since detection of neuroblastoma cells in the marrow confirms the diagnosis and also establishes a stage IV disease with its obvious implications. The role of fine needle aspiration cytology is confined to establishing a tissue diagnosis in advanced inoperable cases.

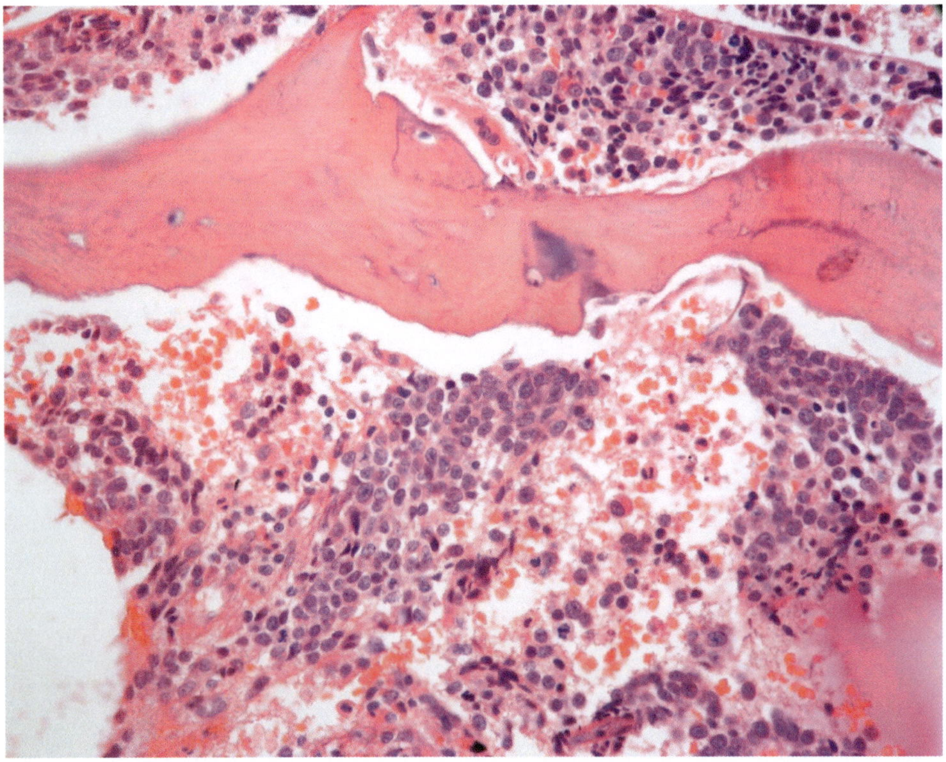

Fig 4.24 Metastatic neuroblastoma in bone marrow: the tumor cells often mistaken for those of acute lymphoblastic leukemia in children

The role of fine needle aspiration cytology is confined to establishing a tissue diagnosis in advanced inoperable cases.

Pathology

Gross

The tumor is usually a smooth, sharply circumscribed oval or round mass about 5-10 cm in diameter and presents soft fleshy tissue with reddish mottling on cut section (Fig. 4.25 A). Some tumors display extensive hemorrhages and cystic degeneration (Fig. 4.25 B). In cases with massive tumor size, its origin from the adrenal gland cannot be assessed. A careful search for calcification, which usually appears as yellowish white streaks or specks, should be made.

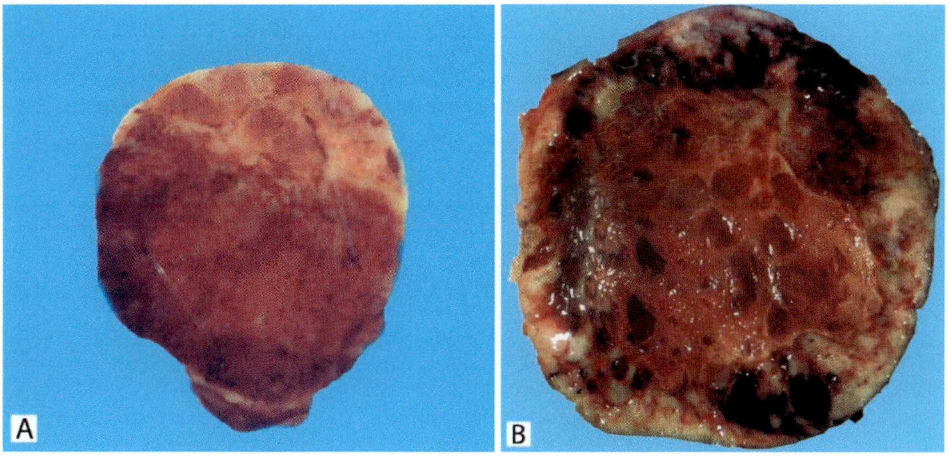

Fig 4.25 Neuroblastoma: (A) a fleshy homogenous reddish encapsulated mass (B) a variegated tumor with cystic degeneration

The tumor cells are small round with no discernible cytoplasm and oval nuclei with salt and paper stippled chromatin. In well-fixed tissue small nucleoli may be seen. Surprisingly nuclear pleomorphism is not present in this primitive and aggressive tumor. The cells are arranged in nests, sheets and masses, which are supported by fibro vascular strands. Three subtypes are recognized:

(i) Undifferentiated subtype exhibits no neuropils or other features of neuroblastic differentiation (Fig. 4.26 A, B). Immunohistochemistry, electron microscopy or molecular methods may be required to arrive at a diagnosis of neuroblastoma in difficult cases.

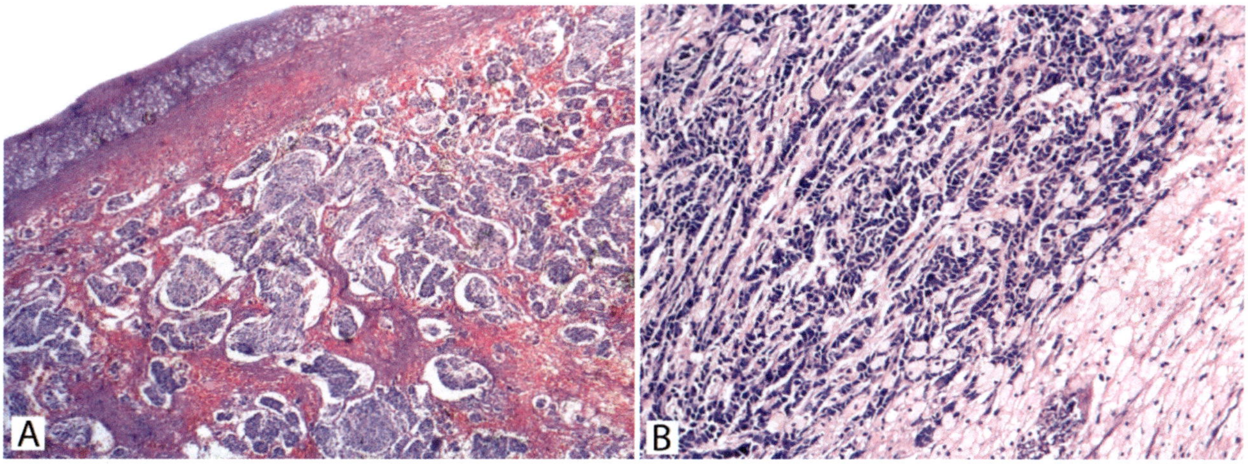

Fig 4.26 Undifferentiated neuroblastoma: (A) small undifferentiated cells of neuroblastoma in compact nests separated by vascular fibrous septa, compressed adrenal gland seen at the periphery; (B) undifferentiated neuroblastoma with no rosette or neuropil

(ii) Poorly differentiated subtype shows good evidence of neuroblastic differentiation in the form Homer-Wright Rosettes and neuropil in the background (Fig.4. 27 A, B, C) Differentiation towards ganglion cells may be present. Differentiating foci should constitute less than 5% of the tumor.

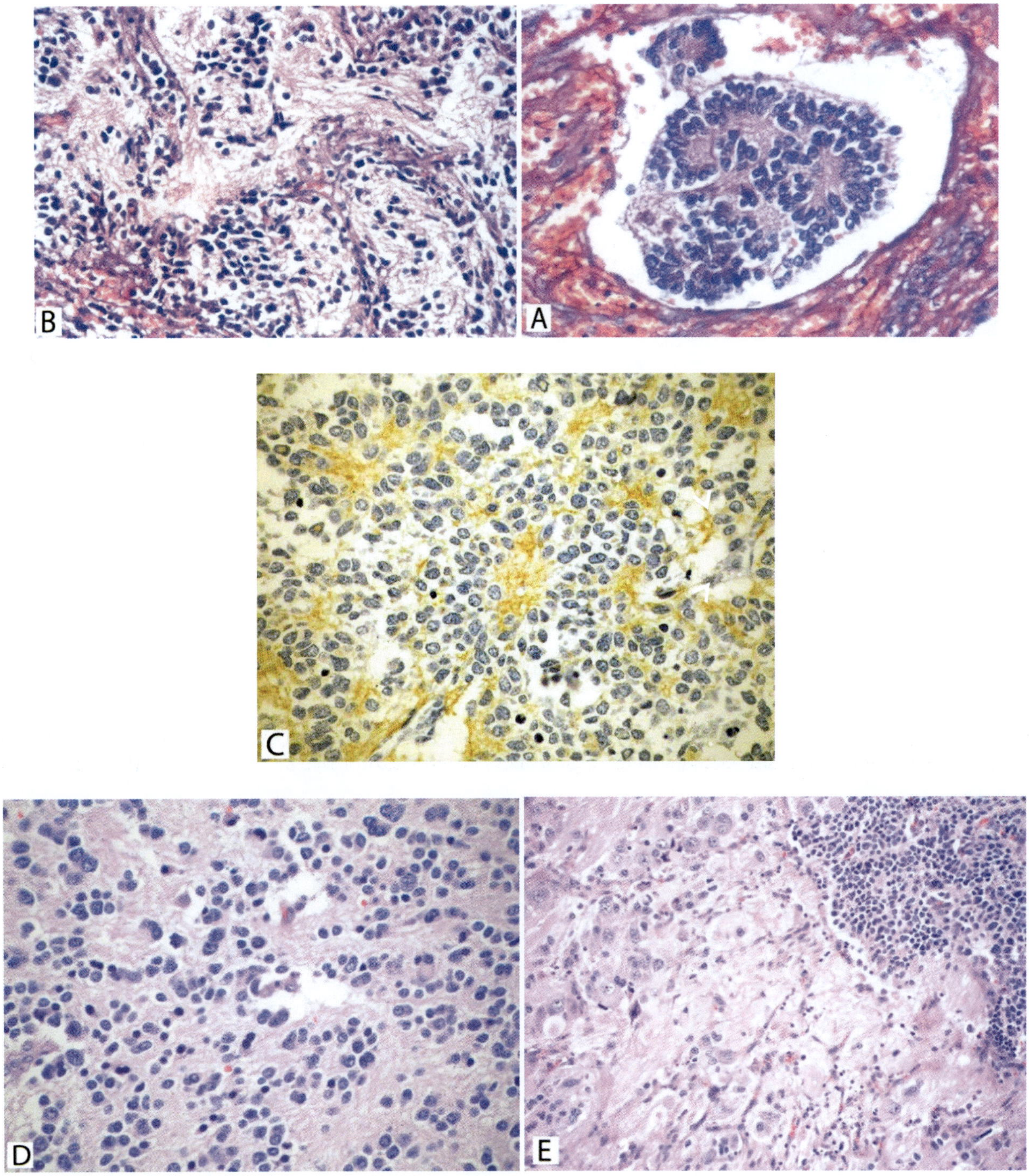

Fig 4.27 Poorly differentiated neuroblastoma: (A) a group of three Homer Wright rosettes almost diagnostic of neuroblastoma; (B) in this field abundant fibrillary matrix or "neuropil" is evident (C) Synaptophysin positive fibrillary material in rosettes; (D) maturing neuroblastoma, large nucleated cells are developing ganglion cells; (E) a nodule of neuroblasts (top right corner) sharply separated from a loose sheet of differentiated ganglion cells

(iii) Differentiating subtype is a neuropil predominant tumor that has several foci (>5%) of ganglionic differentiation (Fig. 4.27 D, E). It can be substantial but never form more than 50% of the tumor. Some Schwannian stroma is always present

Immunohistochemistry

Immunostains for neuron specific enolase (NSE), synaptophysin (Fig. 4.27 C) and chromogranin are all employed for demonstration of neuronal differentiation. The latter two reagents are more reliable than staining for NSE, which is sensitive but less specific.(76, 77, 78).

Electron Microscopy

Neuroblastoma will show neuritic processes containing array of microtubules and membrane bound electron dense core granules (Fig. 4.28 A, B) which are pathognomonic of neuroblastoma (79). In other neuronal or neuroectodermal tumors (PNET) the granules are sparsely populated and of uneven size and the neuritic processes are ill defined. The small cell rhabdomyosarcoma can be readily identified by demonstration of actin and myosin filaments in the cytoplasm.

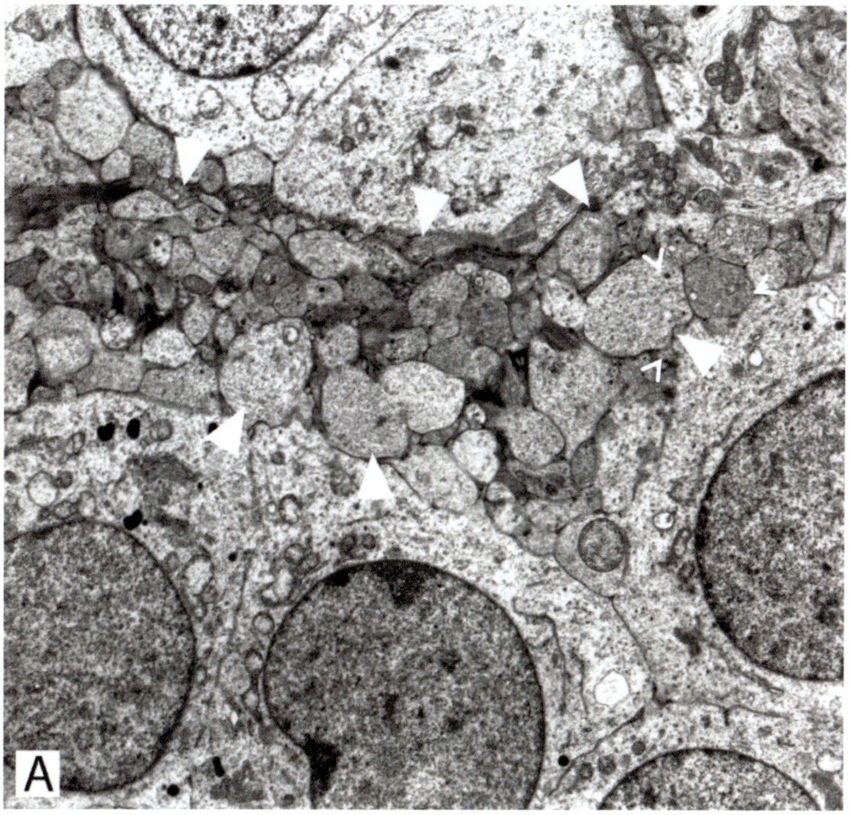

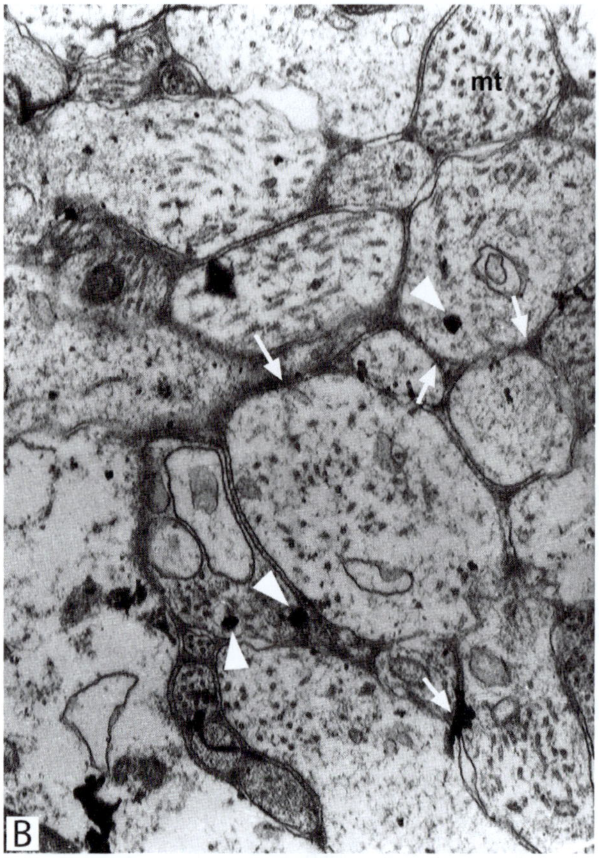

Fig 4.28 Ultrastructure of neuroblastoma: (A) A poorly differentiated neuroblastoma with a neuropil in the center (arrow heads); (B) cell processes rich in microtubules and synaptic junctions (white arrows), an occasional dense core neuroendocrine granule (white arrowheads)

Ganglioneuroblastoma (Schwannian stroma-rich tumors)

Ganglioneuroblastoma is a more differentiated form of neuroblastoma and is considered to arise through a process of maturation from an antecedent neuroblastoma, although this cannot be proved in most cases. Majority is encountered in children, but examples in adult have been reported. Most ganglioneuroblastomas are located in the retroperitoneum and mediastinum rather than the adrenal gland. We have encountered one example in neck, one in the mediastinum and only one in the adrenal gland. Grossly, these tumors are firm, grey white with few relatively soft hemorrhagic areas and calcification (Fig.4.29 A, B, C).

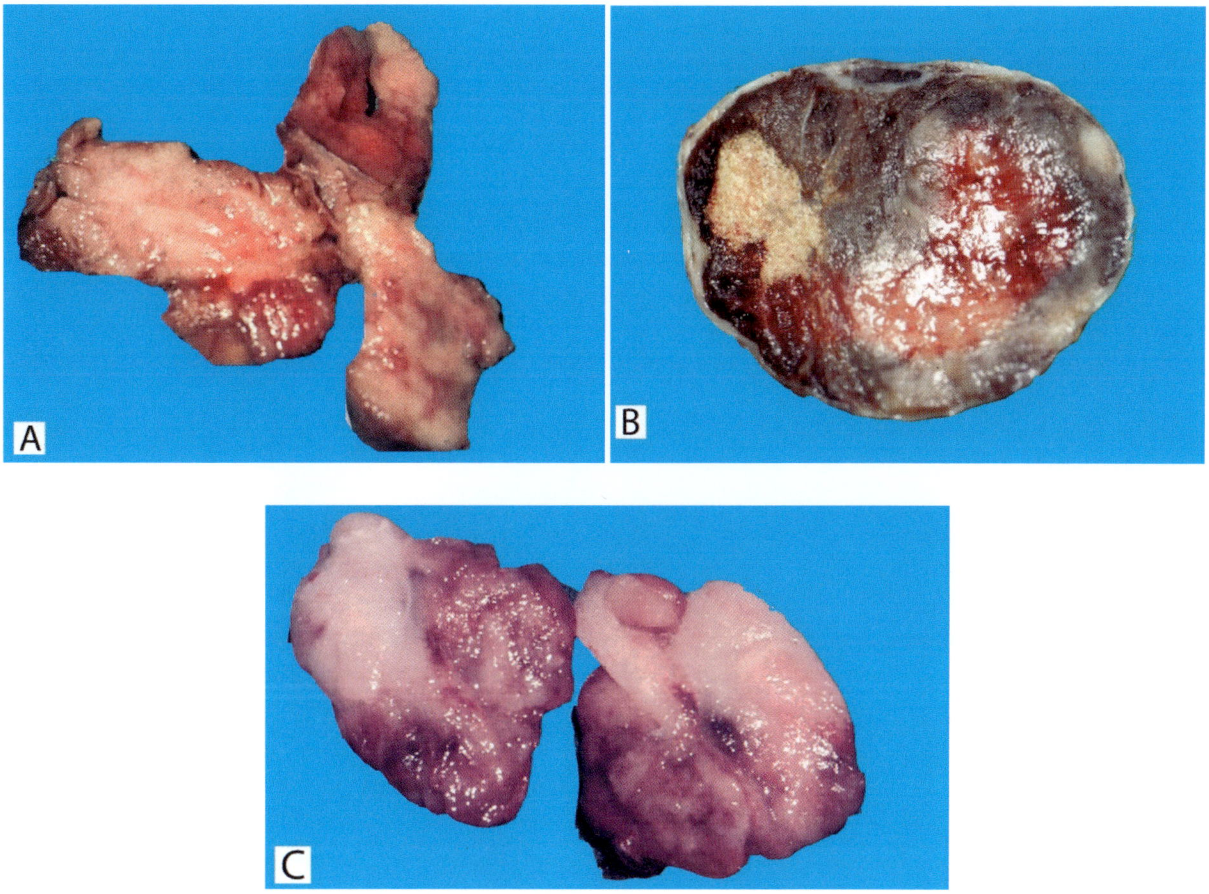

Fig 4.29 Ganglioneuroblastoma: (A) tumor in the neck of an 8 year old boy, evidently arose from cervical sympathetic chain; (B) tumor of adrenal gland in a 14 year old girl, pale yellowish patch of calcification (at upper left) seen in other wise reddish brown encapsulated mass; (C) the lobulated fleshy reddish white tumor was excised from posterior mediastinum

Two histological patterns are recognized, intermixed (Fig. 4.30A, B) and nodular (Fig. 4.30 C). In the more common intermixed pattern, there is an intimate mixture of small round darkly staining neuroblasts, cells with intermediate differentiation and well-formed ganglion cells in a background rich in fine fibrillar network. The tumor shows cells in various stages of differentiation towards ganglion cells. In addition, a variable number of spindly Schwann cells in fascicles or sheets are present and these constitute the "stroma. The ultrastructure shows well developed neuroblasts with microtubules and dense core membrane bound granules (Fig. 4.30 D)

The nodular or composite form shows macroscopically visible nodules of neuroblastoma with an abrupt zone of transition between the nodule and the Schwannian stroma-rich background. This type of ganglioneuroblastoma is more aggressive than the other type.

In general, ganglioneuroblastoma enjoys much better prognosis than neuroblastoma.

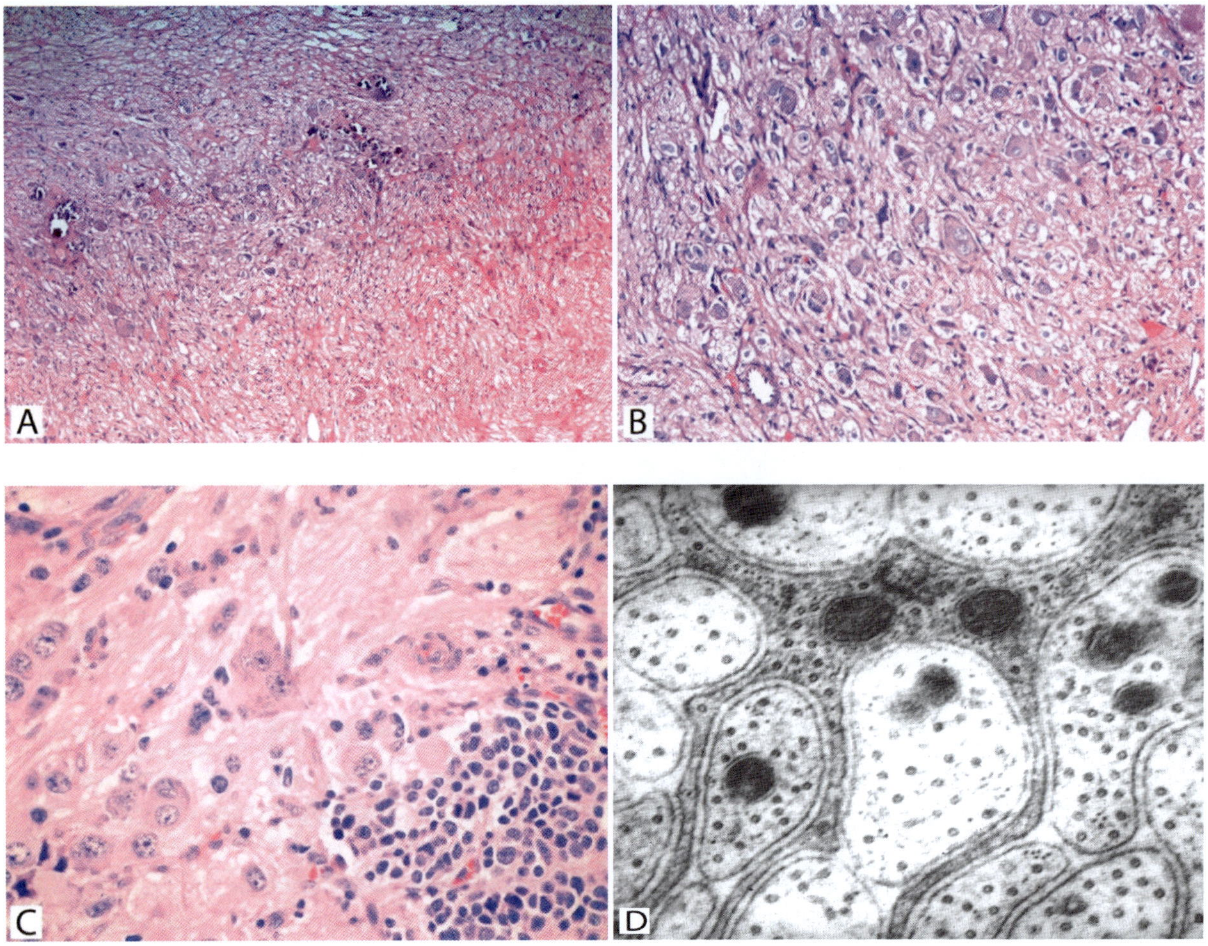

Fig 4.30 Ganglioneuroblastoma: (A) scattered ganglion cells intimately mixed with small undifferentiated cells and spindly stroma; (B) high power view of ganglion cells and spindly cells (Schwann cells); (C) a nodule of neuroblasts and well defined population of mature ganglion cells; (D) processes of ganglion cells rich in microtubules and dense core granules

Ganglioneuroma

This is the most completely differentiated member of neuroblastoma group and is always benign. It characteristically occurs in older patients, and in adults constitutes the most common tumor of sympathetic system. The tumor is often very bulky, well encapsulated and composed of rubbery firm whitish or gray white tissue (Fig. 4.31 A.B. C).

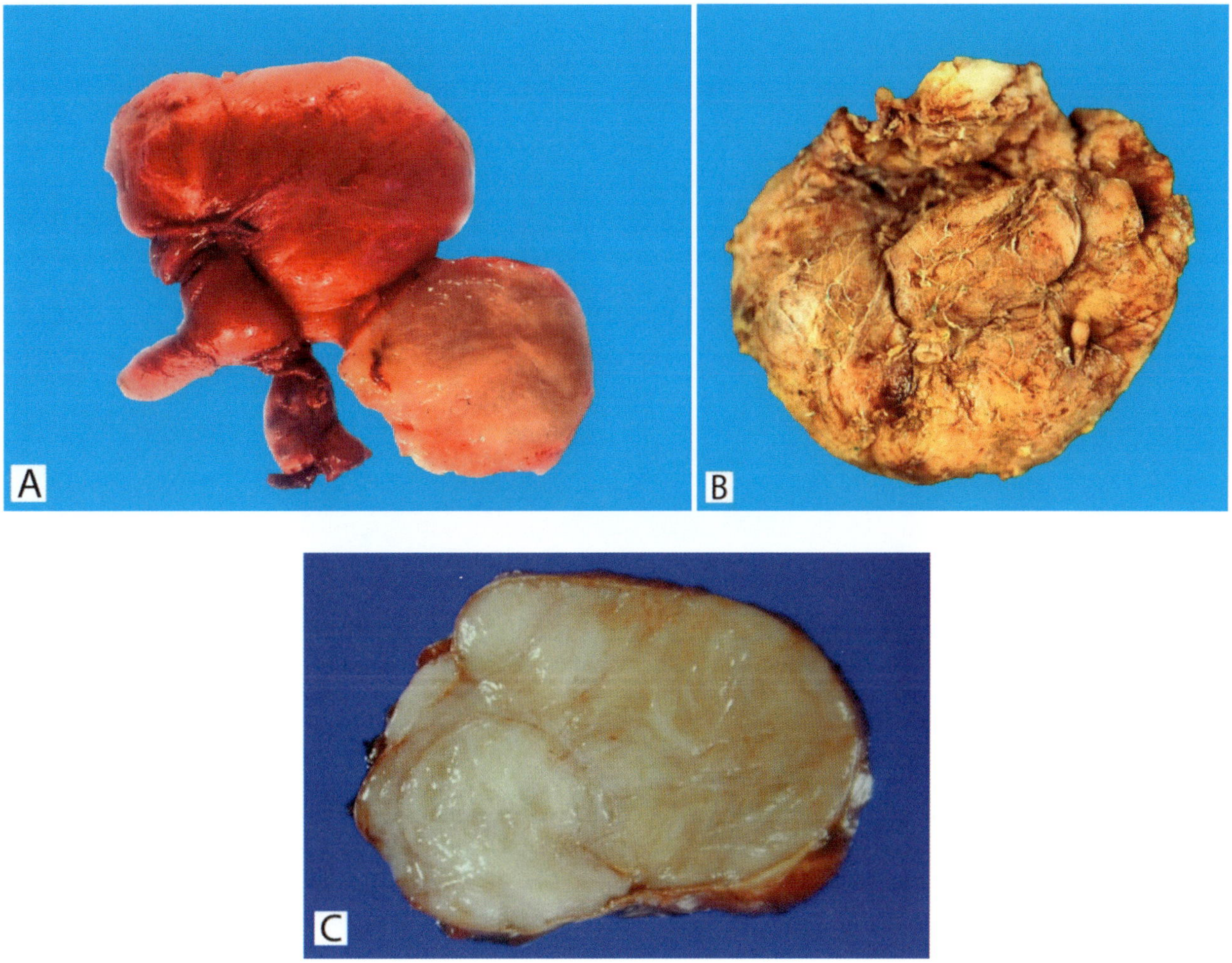

Fig 4.31 Ganglioneuromas: (A) large bilobed encapsulated tumor in close contact with uterus; (B) large encapsulated bilobed nodular mass (455 g) from retroperitoneal region; (C) well encapsulated lobulated focally translucent grey white tumor excised from adrenal gland in a 20 year old man

This is the most differentiated form of neuroblastic tumor. It is composed of large tracts of Schwannian stroma and fully differentiated ganglion cells. Non-differentiating neuroblastic cells are absent. The mature subtype shows Schwannian and neuritic stroma with admixed fully mature ganglion cells.

Histologically it appears like a neurofibroma with the exception of the presence of loose groups of large but mature ganglion cells. (Fig. 4.32 A, B). Posterior mediastinum is the most frequent location followed by retroperitoneum. Immunohistochemistry and electron microscopy are not required for diagnosis. The electron photomicrographs (Fig. 4.32 C, D) reveal a ganglion cell and a Schwannian component

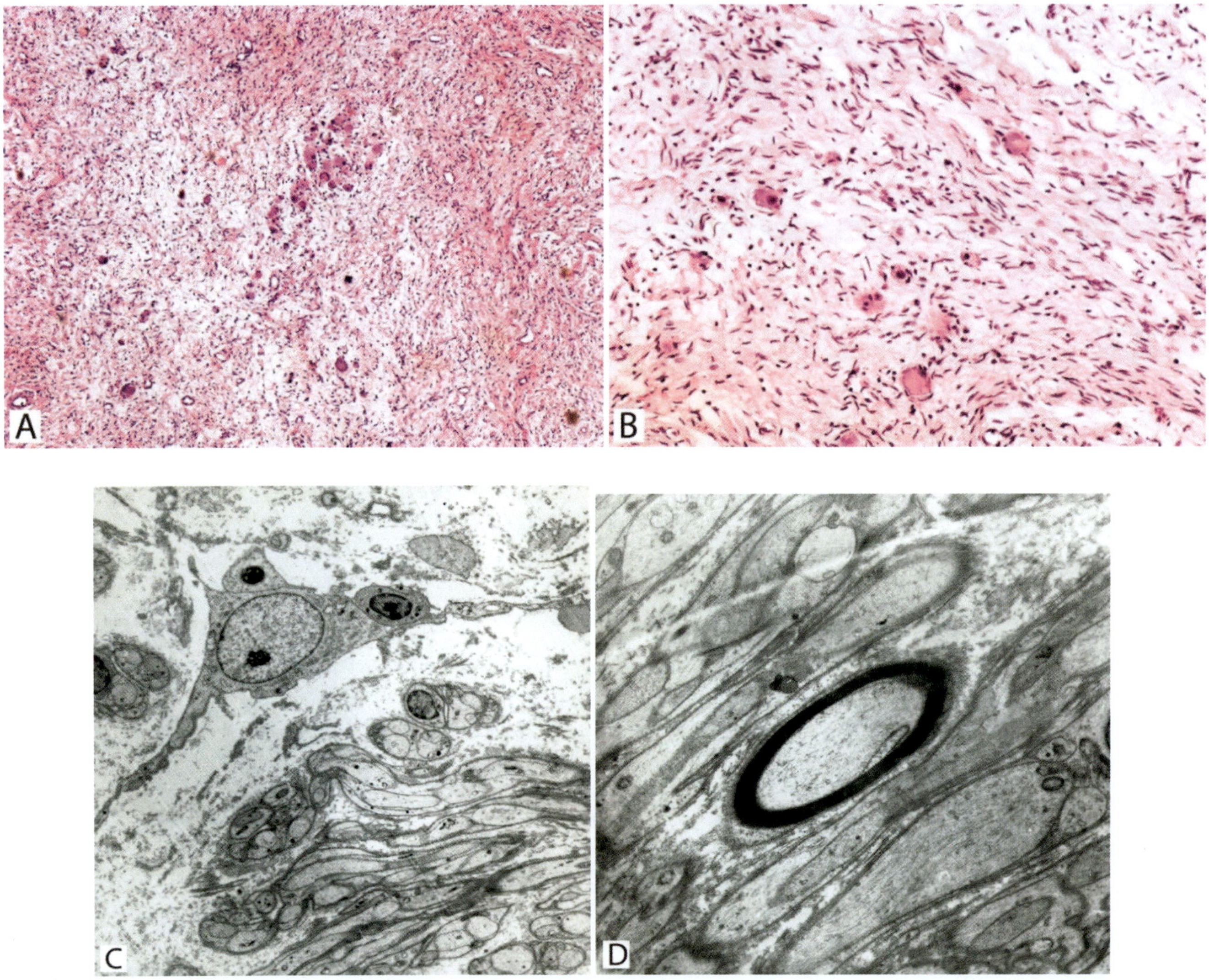

Fig 4.32 Ganglioneuroma: (A, B) loose groups of well formed ganglion cells and abundant Schwannian stroma; (C) Triangular shaped ganglion cell and Schwannian component with large cluster of axons (lower right); (D) higher power of above: a fascicle of axons (one myelinated) coated with basal lamina seen.

Neuroblastoma in children over 5 years of age, adolescents and adults

Neuroblastoma in children over 5 years of age and adolescents are uncommon, display an aggressive behavior and less favorable prognosis compared to neuroblastoma in children under 5 years of age (80). Occurrence of neuroblastoma in adults ("adult neuroblastoma") is indeed rare and in one literature review only 60 cases of adult neuroblastoma have been reported as of 2007 (81). It is difficult to assess the validity of this diagnosis in the era prior to demonstration of the diagnostic translocations in cases of ES/PNET. The diagnosis was always based on histological findings, ultrastructural demonstration of neurites with granules and tubules and expression of synaptophysin and chromogranin on immunohistochemistry. However, demonstration of excess catecholamine excretion (urinary Vanillylmandelic Acid (VMA) testing), which is characteristic of neuroblastoma, is acceptable for diagnosis of adult neuroblastoma even without the molecular confirmation. In one series of adult neuroblastoma, excess catecholamine excretion was reported in 9 out of 27 cases (82).

Differential Diagnosis of Neuroblastoma and Other Small Blue Cell Tumors **(83-91)**

The tumor cells of a neuroblastoma are often indistinguishable from other small cell malignant tumors such as Ewing's sarcoma, lymphoma, alveolar rhabdomyosarcoma etc. Neuroblastoma in adrenal gland with elevated catecholamine levels and characteristic morphology poses no diagnostic problem. However, extra-adrenal neuroblastoma occurring in sympathetic chain will have to be differentiated from a host of undifferentiated small blue cell tumors, which include:

1) Ewing's sarcoma / Primitive neuroectodermal tumor (PNET) of bones and soft tissues
2) Askin Tumor (thoraco-pulmonary small round cell tumor - PNET)
3) Non Hodgkin lymphoma (lymphoblastic)
4) Embryonal/alveolar rhabdomyosarcoma
5) Desmoplastic small round cell tumor
6) Anaplastic Nephroblastoma (Wilm's tumor) in the appropriate setting
7) Embryonal Hepatoblastoma in the appropriate setting

The subject is of paramount importance from the therapeutic and prognostic point of view.

Ewing's sarcoma (ES) and peripheral primitive neuroectodermal tumors (PNET) are rare sarcomas of bones and soft tissues. Stout described an undifferentiated tumor of ulner nerve, in which round cells formed rosettes and the term peripheral neuroepithelioma was coined. ES and PNET were regarded as separate entities for many years. The distinction blurred when Angervall and Enzinger (84) reported "extra-skeletal neoplasm resembling Ewing's sarcoma" and Jaffe et al (1984) described "the neuroectodermal tumor of bone". It was subsequently established that both ES & PNET share a balanced translocation (11:22) (q24:q12) in 90% of cases. Very few laboratories have facilities for molecular testing and now immunohistochemical staining for FLI-1 protein is available. It is positive in more than 70% cases of ES/PNET. The central primitive neuroectodermal tumors and olfactory neuroblastoma (Esthesioneuroblastoma) have not been included in ES/PNET because of absence of CD 99 expression and ES/PNET translocations.

As sympathetic chain is distributed widely in paravertebral region, neuroblastomas arising in these locations are difficult to differentiate from soft tissue Ewing's tumor / PNET and other small round cell tumors (Fig. 4.33 A). In vast majority of cases, glycogen (Fig.4. 33 B) is present in the cytoplasm but it is also seen in lymphoma cells and cells of embryonal rhabdomyosarcoma, and hence not specific. Panel of immunohistochemistry using stains for MIC2 (CD99), Fli1, LCA, cytokeratin, desmin, Myo-D1, myogenin, TEL1, EMA, synaptophysin, chromogranin are quite reliable in arriving at the diagnosis of ES/PNET. CD99 is usually negative in neuroblastomas. (Fig. 4.33 C). Molecular signatures for small round cell tumors are diagnostically the most conclusive e.g. Flurescent in-situ hybridization (FISH) study for EWSR1 break-apart for Ewing's sarcoma/PNET; n-myc FISH / chromogenic in-situ hybridization testing to detect amplification in neuroblastoma. Our experience of extra-adrenal neuroblastoma group of tumors is compiled in Table 4.4.

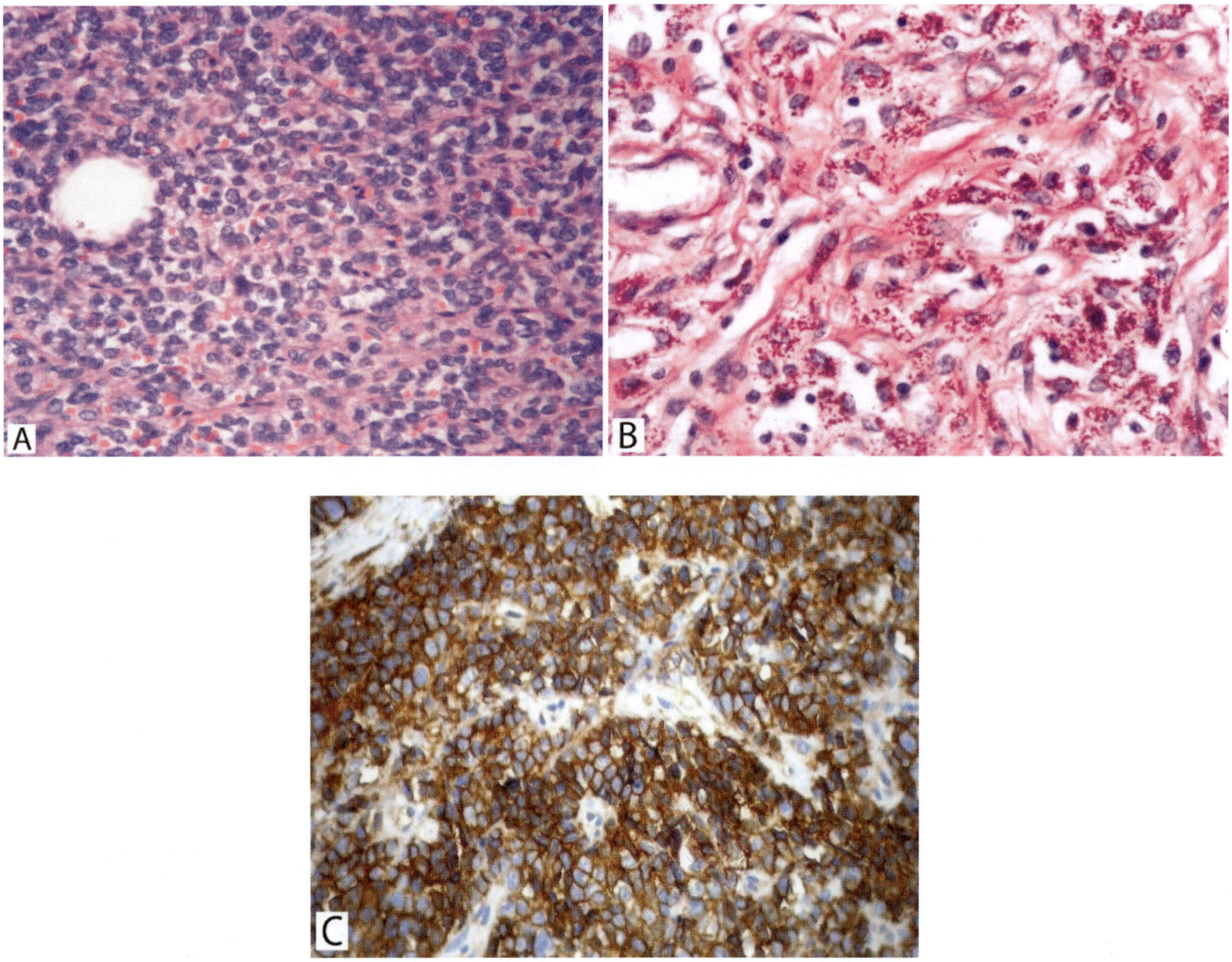

Fig 4.33 EWS/PNET: (A) undifferentiated small round cell tumor in paravertebral region; (B) PAS positive glycogen granules (C) MIC2 (CD99) expressed on the cell membranes. Courtesy: Dr. Anita Borges, Raheja hospital, Mumbai, India

Table 4.4 Extra-adrenal Neuroblastoma Group (N=30) Author's Series 1970-2006)	
Neuroblastoma (16)	
Cervical	2
Mediastinal	5
Abdominal	9
Ganglioneuroblastoma (6)	
Cervical	1
Mediastinal	2
Abdominal	3
Ganglioneuoma (8)	
Mediastinal	2
Retroperitoneal	6

Grading of neuroblastoma

Histological grading in neuroblastoma is a difficult exercise and has limited prognostic significance. Age of the patient, location of the tumor and stage of the disease are the most important factors influencing survival. Most of the grading systems have been difficult to implement because of lack of reproducibility. Differentiation in neuroblastoma refers to the nature of the supporting stroma and the proportion of ganglion cell elements. (92, 93). According to some studies any histological differentiation such as presence of neurofibrillary intercellular material or rosettes is indicative of better prognosis (94, 95).

Table 4.5: International Neuroblastoma Pathology Classification: Subtypes (96)	
Neuroblastoma (Schwannian stroma-poor)	
	Undifferentiated subtype
	Poorly differentiated subtype
	Differentiated subtype
Ganglioneuroblastoma (Schwannian stroma-rich)	
	Intermixed
	Nodular
Ganglioneuroma (Schwannian stroma-rich)	
	Maturing subtype
	Mature subtype

Table 4.6: International Neuroblastoma Pathology Classification (96)		
Age	Favorable Histology	Unfavorable Histology
Any	Ganglioneuroma intermixed Ganglioneuroblastoma-nodular*	Ganglioneuroblastoma-nodular* Neuroblastoma-undifferentiated
< 1.5 years	Neuroblastoma-poorly differentiated with low or intermediate MKI	Neuroblastoma- With high MKI
1.5 years to <5 years	Neuroblastoma-poorly differentiating with low MKI	Neuroblastoma- poorly differentiated, any MKI Neuroblastoma-differentiating with intermediate or high MKI
>5 years	-	Neuroblastoma-Any subtype and any MKI

Tables 5 and 6: tabulated salient points obtained from data of (Reference 96) Shimada H, Ambros IM, Dehner LP, et al. The International Neuroblastoma Pathology Classification (The Shimada System) Cancer 86:364, 1999

Is it worth classifying neuroblastoma by a system as complex as the INPC? The answer is yes. Several studies have confirmed its prognostic value. Many of the neuroblastoma risk group schemes use this classification as one of the parameters in assigning patients to the low intermediate or high risk categories. These risk categories, which always include parameters such as age and stage, may also include markers such as ploidy and MYCN status, 17q gain, LOH at 11q, 14qand 1p, and expression of TRK A, B, C. The value of prognostic groupings is in assigning appropriate treatment to patients and standardizing parameters for clinical trials.

Stage

The most frequently used staging system has been the one developed by Evans et al (97):

I Tumor confined to organ of origin

II Tumor extending beyond the site of origin but not crossing midline; nodes on same side may be involved.

III Tumor extending beyond the midline (Fig.4. 34); nodes on both sides may be involved

IV Metastatic disease involving organs, bones, soft tissues, distant nodes

IVS Otherwise stage I or II disease but with metastases confined to liver, bone marrow or skin

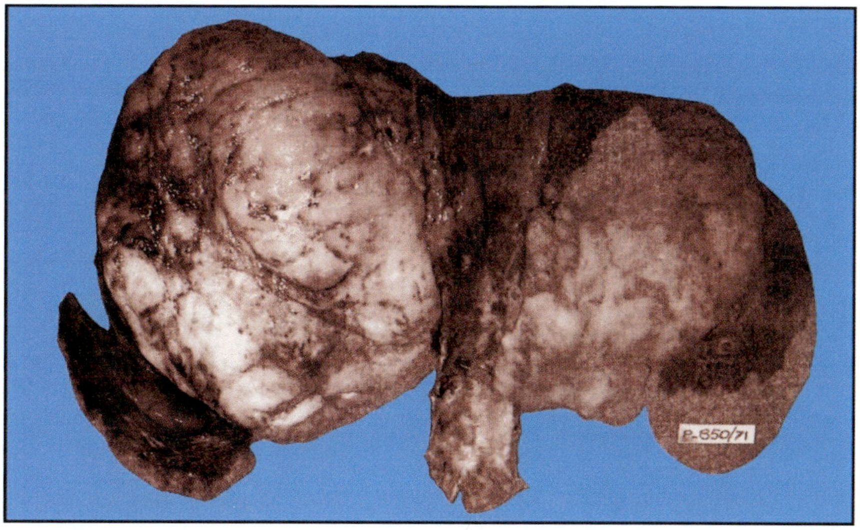

Fig 4.34 A huge neuroblastoma: on both sides of the aorta, seen at autopsy

In stage IVS, 'S' stands for special and the uniqueness lies in complete regression of such a disseminated disease even without treatment. In fact most such patients are better off without chemotherapy.

The clinical stage is up staged when operative and pathological findings are available. Carlsen et al (97 A) analyzed 253 cases of retrospectively staged children and concluded that Evans staging (97 A) was the best prognostic system among 8 different systems evaluated.

Prognosis

The ultimate outcome in this very enigmatic childhood cancer is governed by multiple factors.

1. Age: As a prognostic variable, age at diagnosis of neuroblastoma surpasses all other features including grades and stage in its impact on survival. An overall 90% long term survival is expected in children under 1 year age. This is true even in stage IV cases under 1 year age. The outlook in older children and those with 'adult neuroblastoma' is dismal.
2. Stage: The two year disease free survival is 95-100 for stage I, 85-90% stage II, 50-60% stage III, 10-15% stage IV, and 60-65% stage IV S (68).
3. Site of primary tumor: Children with mediastinal neuroblastoma fare much better than those with abdominal primary, principally because of early appearance of symptoms and early diagnosis before development of metastasis in the former.
4. Neuron specific enolase: The protein is expressed by neuroblastoma cells and is elevated in the serum in advanced cases. Zeltzer et al (98) found than serum levels of NSE 100 ng/ml or more are associated with poor disease free survival and that NSE serum levels were much lower in stage IV S.
5. Serum ferritin levels: Levels above 140 ng/ml are encountered in advanced neuroblastoma. In infants with neuroblastoma in stages I, II and IVS, serum ferritin values are normal. Survival rates were high among those with normal serum ferritin (99, 100).
6. N-MYC oncogene activation: The N-MYC gene is normally present as a single diploid copy in the normal genome and is expressed in many other tumors. However, in advanced stages of neuroblastoma, multiple copies of N-MYC gene are present. This gene amplification is an indicator of poor prognosis and in stage I, II and IVS only single copy of the gene is present. Gene amplification refers to neuroblastoma cells having homogenous staining regions on chromosomes of extra chromosomal double minutes (acentromeric chromatin bits) (101).

In conclusion, the prognosis in neuroblastoma is excellent in the case of the following:

i) Infant under 1 year of age

ii) Low level of serum NSE
iii) Normal serum ferritin
iv) Presence of single copy of N-MYC gene
This information is very useful in determining the duration and intensity of chemotherapy

Pheochromocytoma

Tumor of chromaffin cells of the adrenal gland and autonomous nervous system are called pheochromocytoma or paraganglioma. Traditionally pheochromocytoma has been considered as chromaffin and paraganglioma as non-chromaffin on the basis of strong positive staining with dichromate salts in the former and negative staining with the latter. Now it is recognized that both are derived from the same cell and are morphologically identical. However, by convention, the term pheochromocytoma has been restricted to tumors arising within adrenal medulla and this lesion is often associated with excess catecholamine secretions and hypertension.

The tumors arising in Jugulo-tympanic (glomus jugulare), carotid bony (carotid body tumor), aortic arch ganglia, etc. are called paragangliomas or chemodectomas. Now, the latter term is used only for carotid body and aortic body tumors. The paragangliomas do show catecholamines in tissues but are functionally inactive,

Incidence

Pheochromocytoma is a rare tumor. We have encountered 117 cases of pheochromocytoma in the last 20 years from 6 institutions. During the same period of time 11 cases of paragangliomas have been encountered in the neck and retroperitoneal region. Two cases of pheochromocytoma with hypertension have been seen in urinary bladder. Some pheochromocytomas are nonfunctioning. In the past, many functional ones remained clinically unsuspected and the reported incidence was as high as 34%, discovered at surgery or autopsy (102). With increasing awareness of this lesion and ease with which detection is possible with biochemical and imaging techniques assistance, autopsy incidence has dropped.

Significantly, it needs to be stressed that the incidence of multicentricity in pheochromocytomas is as high as 10% and this has obvious therapeutic implications.

Clinical findings

Pheochromocytomas are most common in 4th and 5th decade of life with mean age of 45.5 years (range 12 to 80 years) (103). Pheochromocytoma is often referred to as a 10% tumor, because 10% are malignant, 10% bilateral, 10% extra-adrenal and 10% occur in children. Other notable clinical manifestations in childhood pheochromocytomas include familial occurrence and association with syndromes like neurofibromatosis, multiple endocrine neoplasia, etc. (104-107).

All signs and symptoms of pheochromocytomas are related to secretion of powerful vasoactive substances, which give rise to either unstable episodic hypertension or sustained hypertension with periods of very severe rise in pressure. A triad of headache, palpitations and sweating in a known hypertensive subject predicts pheochromocytoma with 94% specificity (108). Not all patients present with classical clinical picture and in some, the diagnosis may not be suspected or made for several years. A few pheochromocytomas may also secrete ACTH, somatostatin, calcitonin vasoactive intestinal peptide (VIP), etc. but usually do not give rise to corresponding endocrine manifestations (108).

Pheochromocytoma associated with syndromes: (109, 110)

1. Von Recklinghausen's disease (neurofibromatosis)
2. Multiple endocrine neoplasm (MEN) Type II (Sipple syndrome) Pheochromocytoma + Medullary carcinoma of thyroid + Parathyroid hyperplasia

3. MEN Type III (Gorlin's syndrome) pheochromocytoma + medullary carcinoma of thyroid + mucosal neuromas
4. Von Hippel-Lindau syndrome (cerebello-retinal hemangioblastomatosis)
5. Tuberous sclerosis

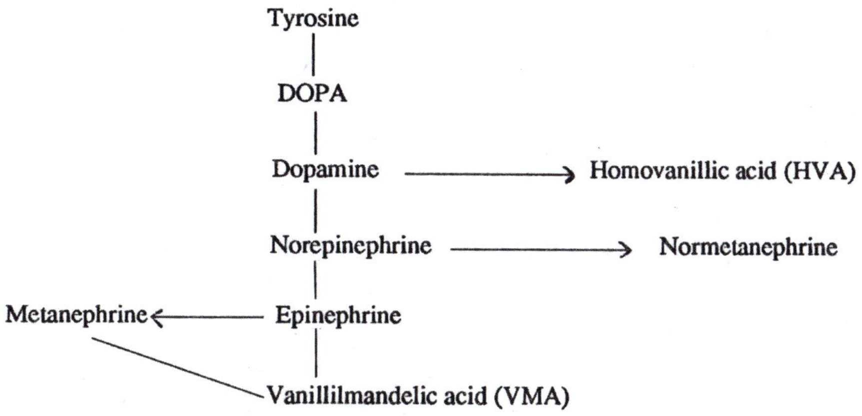

Fig. 4.35 pathways of catecholamine

The diagnosis is made essentially on the demonstration of elevated catecholamines in blood and urine (Fig. 35). Biochemical tests to detect nor epinephrine or epinephrine, metanephrine, nor metanephrine or VMA can be carried out on a 24 hour urinary sample. In the plasma, levels of nor-epinephrine and epinephrine are determined. A value of 2000 pg/ml for NE is diagnostic and values below 500 pg/ml are considered normal.

Radiology:

Once the diagnosis is established, localization of the tumor, adrenal or extra-adrenal, unilateral or bilateral is the next step before surgical treatment. The various techniques include CT scan, MRI, I 131, MIBG scan, and ultrasound.

Gross:

Pheochromocytoma usually appears as a well encapsulated tumor measuring from 3 to 6 cm and weighing about 100 g. Remnants of compressed adrenal gland may be detected externally. Sectioned surface shows a somewhat rubbery tan white tumor with focal hemorrhagic mottling or may present overall dusky red color (Fig. 36 A). Hemorrhages, necrosis and cystic degeneration (Fig. 4.36 B) are found in the more bulky tumors. Rarely, one encounters an almost totally cystic tumor (Fig. 4.36 C) . Infiltration into the surrounding organs or invasion up the inferior vena cava is almost never reported. The tumor tissue turns dark mahogany brown when freshly immersed in dichromate solution at pH 5 to 6 and formalin fixation beings about a brownish black discoloration (Fig.36 D). In our experience these gross findings are found in virtually all samples of pheochromocytoma.

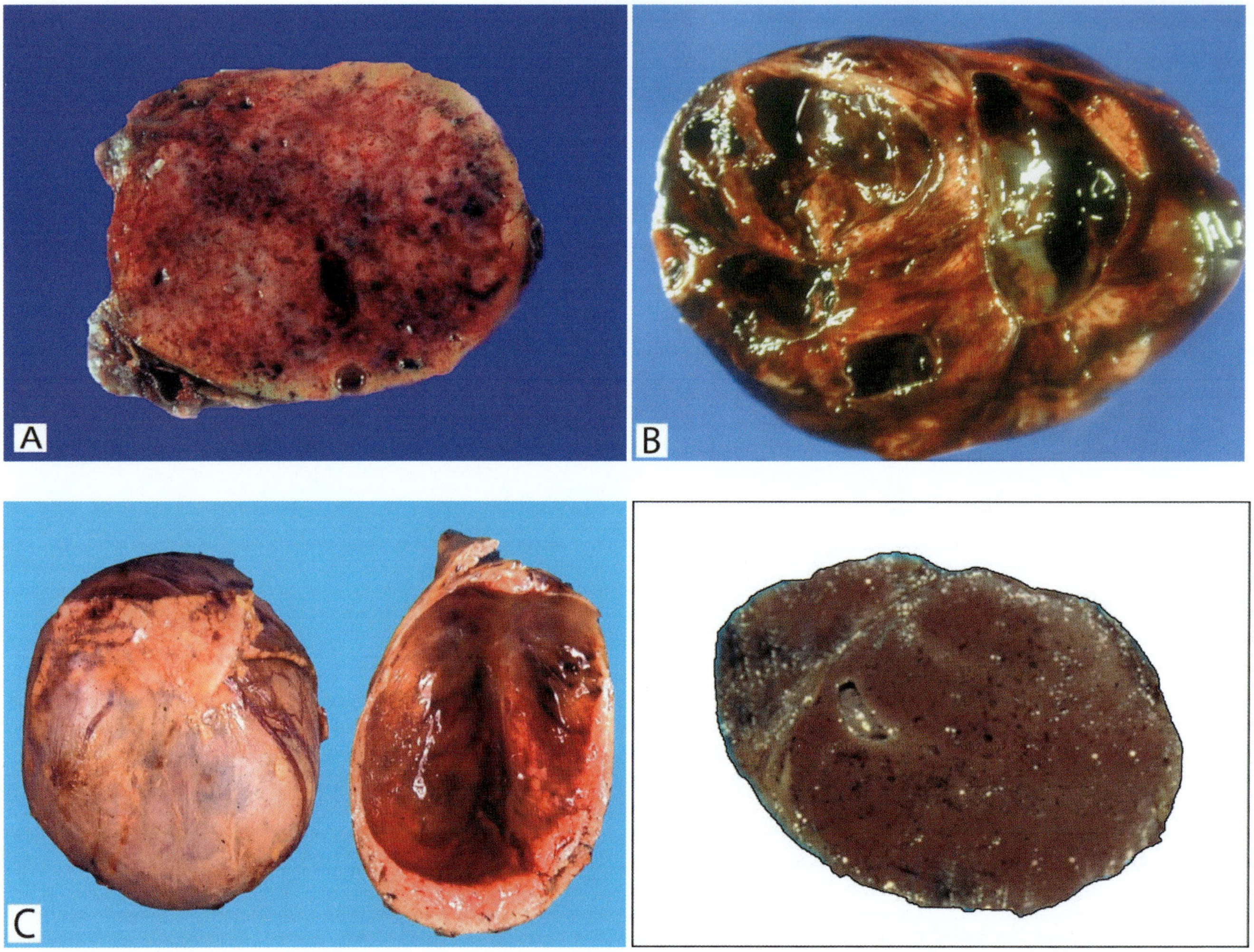

Fig 4.36 Pheochrocytoma: (A) reddish grey tumor with hemorrhagic mottling, compressed adrenal seen at lower left corner; (B) large oval encapsulated reddish tumor with focal cystic degeneration; (C) a completely cystic form of Pheochromocytoma; (D) pheochromocytoma fixed in formalin appears grey black

Hemorrhages, necrosis and cystic degeneration (Fig.4. 36 B) are found in the more bulky tumors. Rarely, one encounters an almost totally cystic tumor (Fig. 4.36C). Infiltration into the surrounding organs or invasion up the inferior vena cava is almost never reported. The tumor tissue turns dark mahogany brown when freshly immersed in dichromate solution at pH 5 to 6 and formalin fixation beings about a brownish black discoloration (Fig.4.36 D). In our experience these gross findings are found in virtually all samples of pheochromocytoma.

Microscopy:

The histological appearance is quite characteristic and the cells are arranged in anastomosing cords and trabeculae or in solid alveolar (zellballen) nesting patterns supported by a delicate rich vascular stroma (Fig. 4.37A). In few cases the pattern is more diffuse. The cells are medium large polyhedral with typically indistinct borders and possess granular pale acidophilic cytoplasm. The nuclei are oval or round and sharply defined with scattered coarsely hyperchromatic enlarged forms. Intranuclear inclusions are often seen. It is not uncommon to find very pleomorphic and even bizarre nuclei (Fig.4.37 B) but this is not a feature of malignancy. The characteristic zellballen pattern is not always present and a diffuse cell arrangement cannot be differentiated from malignant epithelial tumors (Fig 4.37 C). The histological diagnosis in non-functioning tumors or paragangliomas can indeed be difficult and ancillary morphological techniques will be necessary.

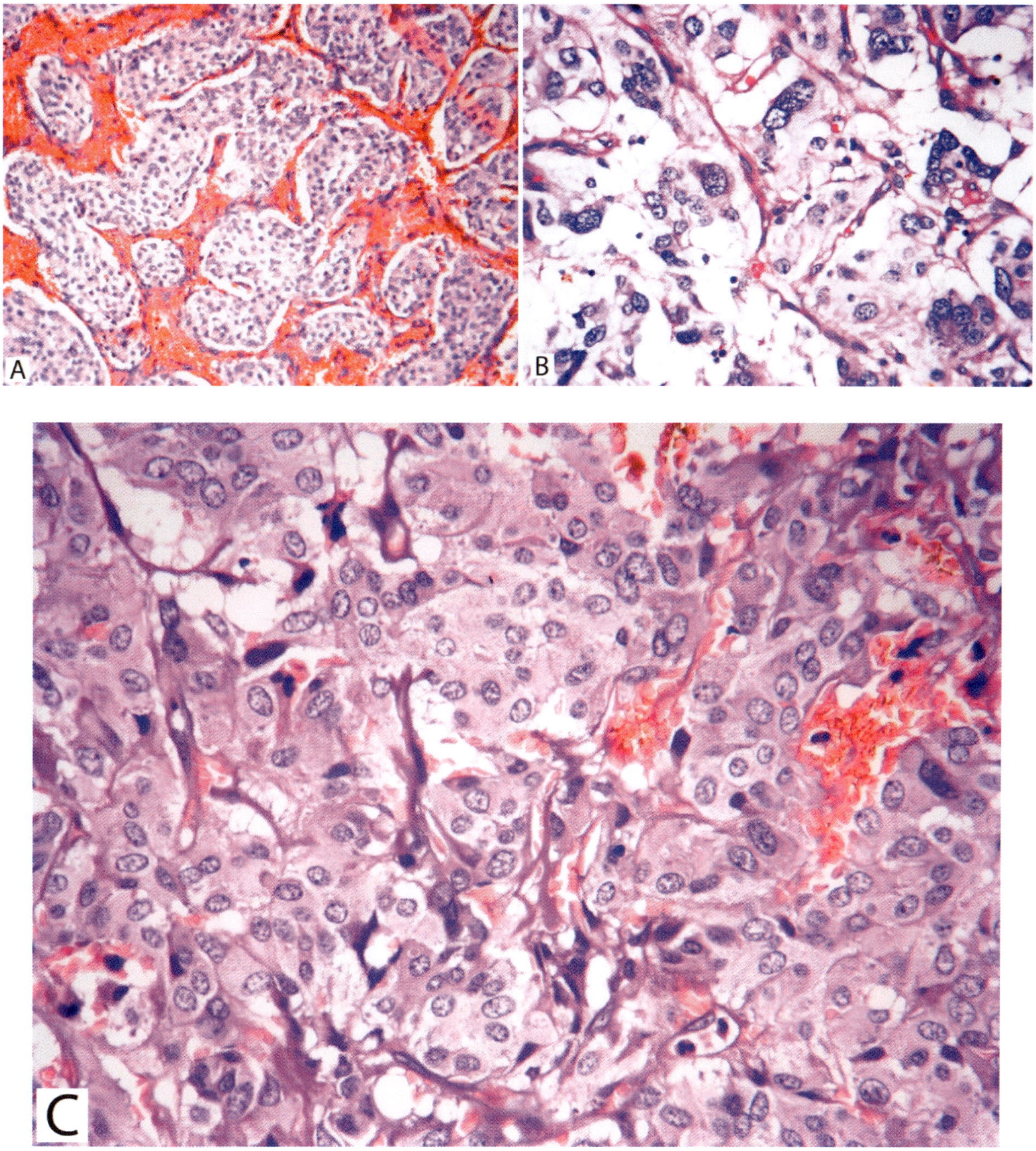

Fig 4.37 Histology of pheochromocytoma: (A) nests of cells ("zellballen") separated by vascular stromal strands; (B) marked nuclear pleomorphism with occasional multinucleated cell; (C) typical zellballen pattern is not seen, differentiation from a carcinoma can be difficult

Postive chromogranin and synaptophysin immunostains and negative cytikeratin are reliable and specific in the diagnosis of pheochromocytoma (Fig. 4.38 A, B). Neuron specific enolase is found in all cases but is less specific. A host of (at least 10) various neuropeptides have been demonstrated in pheochromocytomas. Malignant tumors expressed fewer peptides than benign ones. These findings are surely of interest in understanding the physiology of this unique tumor but such studies are not required for diagnosis. Positive staining with S-100 protein is shown by the sustentacular stromal cells in pheochromocytoma and similar to that in extra-adrenal paraganglioma.

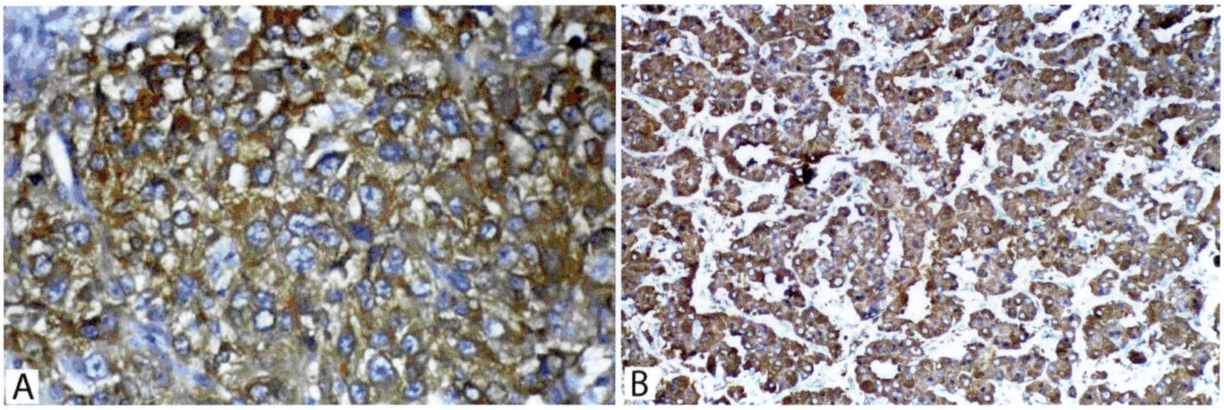

Fig 4.38 Immunohistochemistry: (A) Synaptophysin expressed in the cell cytoplasm; (B) immunostaining for chromogranin strongly positive

Electron microscopy:

The pheochromocytes are endowed with a large population of membrane bound electron dense granules that vary from 150 to 400 nm in size. The larger granules typically show eccentric space and are considered to store norepinephrine. Epinephrine is stored in granules, which possess narrow peripheral halo (Fig. 4.39 A, B). However, according to Medeiros (103) correlation of granule content and morphology is not consistent and reliable.

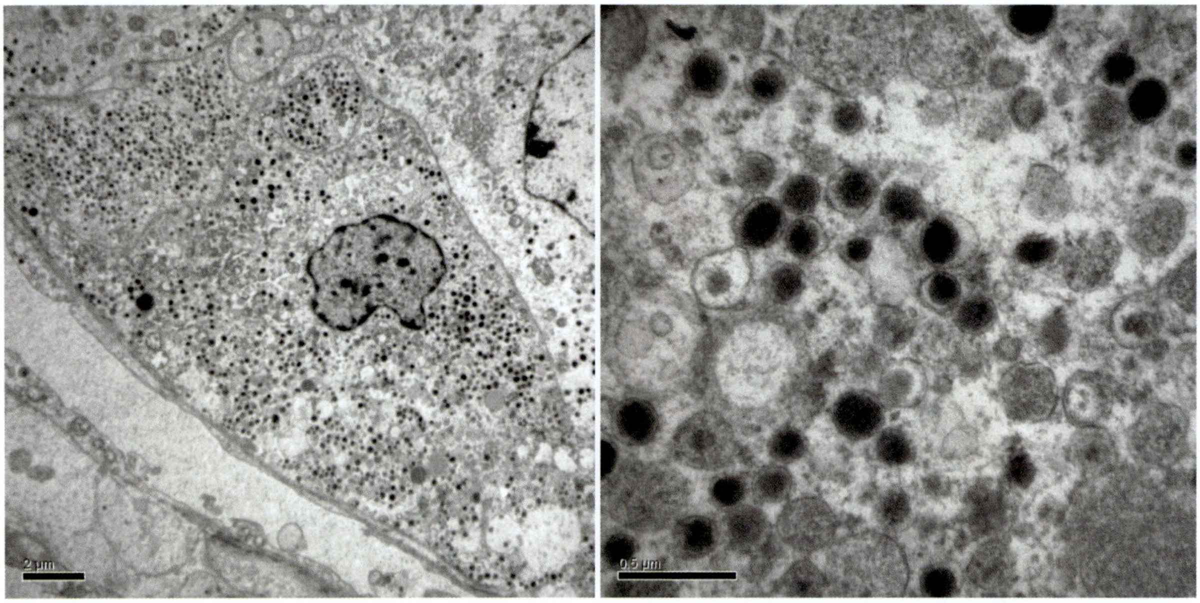

Fig 4.39 Ultrastructure of pheochromocytoma: (A) a richly granulated pheochromocytes; (B) a close up of granules: granules with eccentric halo are known to secrete epinephrine and others nor epinephrine

Malignant Pheochromocytoma

Pheochromocytoma is considered malignant only when metastasis is demonstrated, which implies that conventional morphological criteria of malignancy like mitotic activity, pleomorphism, capsular/and or vascular invasion are unreliable. In our 117 cases of adrenal pheochromocytoma only one was diagnosed as malignant in which a metastatic nodule was found in the duodenal wall. This tumor was identical to all others which exhibited benign behavior. These diagnostic difficulties have given rise to conflicting reports regarding the true incidence of malignant pheochromocytomas. The various studies have quoted an incidence from 7 to 14% of total pheochromocytomas (111-114). Our own experience in this regard is not adequate because of lack of follow up information in some cases.

The situation is similar to that in adrenal cortical carcinomas and criteria like average weight over 100 g. high mitotic count, necrosis, local invasion, vascular invasion have been considered predictive of malignant behavior (108).

Adrenal medullary hyperplasia

This has been established as a clinical entity, in which signs and symptoms suggestive of pheochromocytoma occur and both adrenals show medullary hyperplasia with excess absolute weight of the medullary tissue (Fig. 4.40 A, B). A bilateral or even subtotal adrenalectomy completely relieves the symptoms (115, 116). The sporadic (non-familial) occurrence of adrenal medullary hyperplasia is less common than that reported with multiple endocrine neoplasia type 2, in which it is considered as a precursor lesion for bilateral pheochromocytomas.(117, 118).

One of the earliest manifestations of adrenal medullary hyperfunction in patients with MEN type 2 syndromes is an increased ratio of neither epinephrine to nor epinephrine in urine. The pathological findings in the adrenal glands of 10 patients from large kindred with familial medullary thyroid carcinoma revealed diffuse and multifocal nodular proliferation of adrenal medullary cells. A morphometric analysis based on point counting system was used to assess adrenal medullary volume. It revealed two to three fold increases in medullary volume and weight (118). Adrenal medullary hyperplasia is often misdiagnosed. It is often associated with MEN type 2 syndrome but can also be sporadic. Clinically it is characterized by episodic hypertension and increased catecholamines in plasma and urine (119, 120). In many cases CT/MRI may not reveal adrenal medullary abnormality but MIBG scan is a sensitive and diagnostic imaging modality (121). In one case report, asymptomatic medullary hyperplasia was detected with intraoperative hypertension (122).

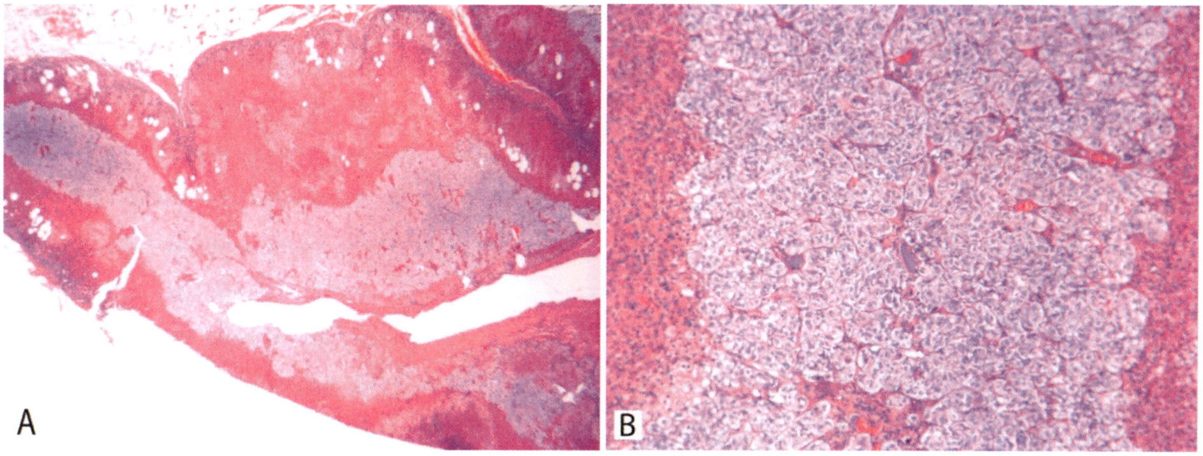

Fig 4.40 Adrenal medullary hyperplasia: (A) medullary cells in compact sheets around adrenal vein, note compressed cortex along inferior margin; (B) high power picture of pale staining adrenal medullary hyperplasia

Pheochromocytoma in hereditary tumor syndromes

A large proportion of pheochromocytomas are sporadic and unilateral. However, about 10% of pheochromocytomas are bilateral and associated with hereditary tumor syndromes. The incidence of familial pheochromocytomas in the reported series' varies from 5% to 11% and has been as high as 31.5 and 46%.(123-127) Neumann, Berger, Sigmund et al (128) studied 82 cases of unselected pheochromocytoma and found that 16 cases (19%) had VHL disease and 3 cases (4%) had MEN 2. The study concluded that all patients with pheochromocytomas should be screened for VHL disease and MEN2 to avert further morbidity and mortality in patients and their families.

The occurrence of familial pheochromocytoma is found to be much higher following a detailed molecular study of patients with familial pheochromocytomas in the last decade. The hereditary tumor syndromes include pheochromocytoma-paraganglioma syndrome (SDHB & SDHD gene) in addition to VHL disease (VHL gene), MEN 2 (RET gene) and neurofibromatosis (Type 1 NF 1 gene) (129-130).

Pheochromocytoma & von Hippel Lindau (VHL) Disease

Von Hippel Lindau (VHL) disease is an autosomal dominant inherited tumor syndrome and germ line mutation in the VHL gene predisposes carriers to tumors in different organs.(133-135). The VHL gene is a tumor suppressor gene and is involved in blood vessels formation. The carriers develop CNS hemangioblastoma, retinal angioma, pheochromocytoma, renal cell carcinoma etc. Recently, Koch et al (136) found that VHL-associated pheochromocytomas had distinct histopathological phenotype as compared with pheochromocytomas in patients with MEN 2. VHL tumors had thick vascular capsule, myxoid and hyalinized stroma, round small to medium tumor cells, predominantly clear cytoplasm, absence of cytoplasmic hyaline globules and lack of nuclear atypia or mitoses.

Pheochromocytoma & Multiple Endocrine Neoplasia type 2 (MEN 2)

Many cases of familial pheochromocytoma occurring in MEN 2 syndromes have been reported. As compared with sporadic pheochromocytomas, the familial ones tend to occur in younger age group. They are more commonly bilateral and frequently associated with other primary neoplasms. MEN syndromes are inherited with an autosomal dominant pattern of inheritance caused by germ line mutations of the RET gene.

MEN type 2a syndrome is the most common form of MEN 2 and is characterized by medullary thyroid carcinoma, pheochromocytoma and parathyroid hyperplasia or adenoma. MEN type 2b is associated with medullary thyroid carcinoma, pheochromocytoma, intestinal ganglioneuromatosis and skeletal deformity. Pheochromocytomas area found in about 50% of patients with MEN 2a and the tumors are bilateral or multifocal in about 60% to 70% (137-139). In MEN 2b, mucosal neuromatous lesions in the gastrointestinal tract often occur at early age and may allow early detection of the disorder. The most important component of MEN 2b is medullary thyroid carcinoma which often pursues an aggressive course with metastases and fatal outcome (140). In both MEN 2 a & 2 b subtypes, pheochromocytoma is an integral part of the syndrome (141).

Pheochromocytoma & Neurofibromatosis (NF 1)

According to Riccardi's estimate the frequency of association of pheochromocytoma in von Recklinghausen neurofibromatosis (NF 1) is less than 1% (142). Walther and others (143) reviewed the literature (total 118 articles) and found that the frequency varied from 0.1% to 5.8%. A total of 148 (M:F = 61:87) cases were clinically identified. The average age was 42 years (1.5 to 74 years). 84% patients had solitary adrenal tumors, 9.6% bilateral and 5.8% ectopic. Symptoms related to pheochromocytoma or hypertension were noted in 78% of the patients and tumors secreted epinephrine and non-epinephrine. 17 out of 148 patients had metastases or local invasion from pheochromocytoma.. It was noted that autopsy incidence of this association was 3.3 % to 13% (144).

Pheochromocytoma & Familial Paraganglioma Syndrome

Germ line mutations of succinic dehydrogenase (SDH) subunits were originally described in hereditary paraganglioma; a dominantly inherited disorder characterized by vascular tumors in the head the neck, most frequently at the carotid bifurcation (145) Germ line mutations of the SDHD, SDHB and SDHC genes are a major cause of hereditary paraganglioma and pheochromocytoma and these genes are classic tumor suppressors. SDHD mutation carriers (PGL-1) had frequent and multifocal head and neck paragangliomas. SDHB mutation carriers (PGL-4), on the other hand, are more likely to develop malignant disease, including renal cell and thyroid carcinomas (146).

Extra-adrenal Sympathetic Paragangliomas

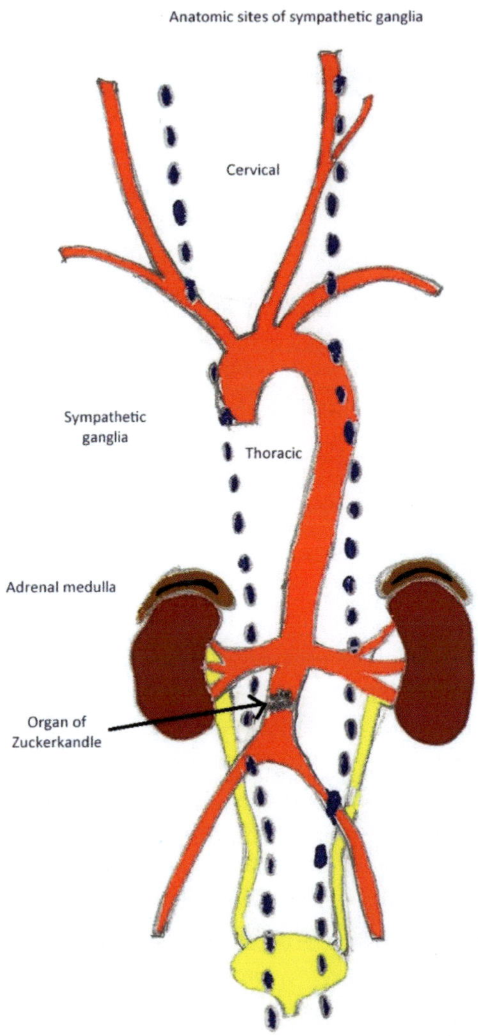

Fig 4.41 Diagram showing sites of sympathetic paragangliomas

Extra-adrenal paraganglia are distributed closely parallel to the sympathetic nervous system in the para-vertebral axis on either side of midline from neck to pelvic floor. Zuckerkandl described extra-adrenal chromaffin tissues, located on either side of the aorta extending from origin of inferior mesenteric artery to just above bifurcation of the aorta. The anatomical distribution of extra-adrenal paragangliomas (Fig 41) is mainly intra-abdominal (85%) This site wise distribution of extra-adrenal paragangliomas varies in different large series'. In Melicow's review of 107 cases, 98% were intra-abdominal, only 2% in neck and thoracic and less than 1% in bladder (147).

Extra-Adrenal Abdominal Paragangliomas:

Majority of intra-abdominal paragangliomas occur in the vicinity of the adrenal gland, renal hilum and organ of Zuckerkandl. They present in 2nd to 3rd decade of life and slight male preponderance is noted. The incidence of patients with signs and symptoms of excess catecholamine secretions is quite high and varies from 25% to 86% in various serises. As a group extra-adrenal paraganglioma tend to be the most aggressive paragangliomas in the sympatho-adrenal system and the rates of malignancy have been variously reported to be 14%, 42% and 50% (148-150). It is important to note that multiple paragangliomas do occur but this should not be construed as evidence of malignancy. Metastasis most frequently occurs in the lymph nodes, bone and liver.

Paragangliomas of Urinary bladder:

Zimmerman reported in 1953, the first of pheochromocytomas arising in the urinary bladder and since then over 100 cases have been reported in the English literature (151). The review of 58 cases (24 AFIP + 34 literature) by Leetsma and Price (152) is the first comprehensive clinico-pathological study on the subject. Males and females are affected with equal frequency, over a wide age range with an average of 41 year (range 11-78 years). Nearly 50% of cases present with triad of episodic hypertension, intermittent hematuria and attack associated with micturition. This clinical presentation is almost pathognomonic of pheochromocytoma of urinary bladder. In this case paraganglioma cells are in sheets, note a fascicle of entrapped bladder muscle (Fig. 4.42A). The diagnosis can be confirmed by measurements of catecholamine and their metabolites in serum and urine. In addition, MIBG scan can readily find the localization of the lesion within the bladder. However, in many cases (nearly 50%) diagnosis of paraganglioma is missed and particularly on TUR specimen a tumor may be reported as transitional cell carcinoma. If characteristic zellballen pattern is seen, suspicion of paraganglioma may arise and the diagnosis can be confirmed on immunohistochemistry (Fig. 4.42 B) and/or electron microscopy.

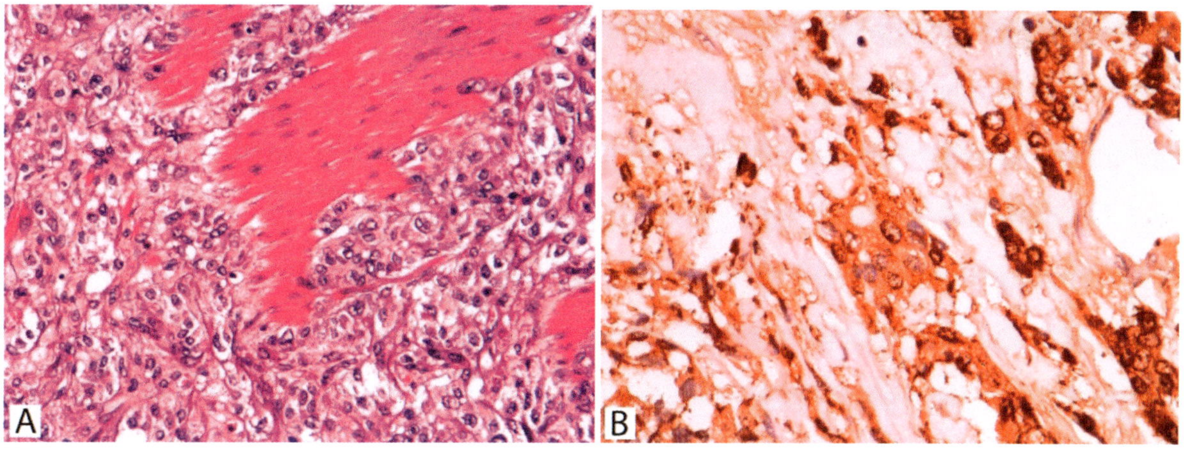

Fig 42 Histology of paraganglioma: (A) Paraganglioma involving bladder muscle; (B) Tumor cells strongly positive for chromogranin immunostaining

The clinical course of bladder paraganglioma is usually benign but in one literature review of 87 patients (183) lymph node metastases were observed in 12 cases (13.8%) and distant metastases in 2 cases (2.3%). As of 2004 (153) up to 180 cases of paraganglioma have been reported of which less than 30 were malignant.

Zhou, Epstein & Young (154) studied 15 cases of paraganglioma of urinary bladder of which 3 were reported as transitional cell carcinoma and 4 only as "bladder tumor" by the referring pathologist. Only 2 cases out of 15 had symptoms suggestive of paraganglioma of bladder. The major histological features that led to misdiagnoses included diffuse growth pattern, focal clear cells, necrosis and muscular invasion with the cautery artifact compounding the diagnostic problem.

Thoracic Paravertebral Paragangliomas

These tumors occur in the posterior mediastinum along the paravertebral sulcus (Fig. 43 A, B) and this will easily distinguish them from aortico-pulmonary paragangliomas that occur in the anterior compartment of the chest. In a review of 31 cases (155), the male to female ratio was almost 2:1, age range 4 months to 67 years with a mean of 29 years and 7% incidence of distant metastases. About 20% of patients had multiple paragangliomas.

Clinically, many paragangliomas at this site present with mass effect, mainly pain or detected incidentally. Many others display signs and symptoms of catecholamine secretion. Odze et al (156) collected 47 cases of posterior mediastinal paragangliomas from the literature and found 6 cases with metastatic disease, 2 of which presented metastatic manifestations ab initio. The case of malignant paraganglioma reported in this paper is reviewed along with 6 cases from the literature and this revealed a male to female ratio of 6:1with a wide range in age at presentation. Two of 7 cases revealed elevated catecholamines with overt functional symptoms in one. On the other hand, 17 of 41 benign cases reported manifestations of excess catecholamine secretions. A study of 12paragangliomas of posterior mediastinum revealed 75% patients alive and well at the end of follow up, one had metastasis to spine and bone marrow and another died of metastases to lymph nodes, lungs and pelvis 14 years after initial diagnosis (157).

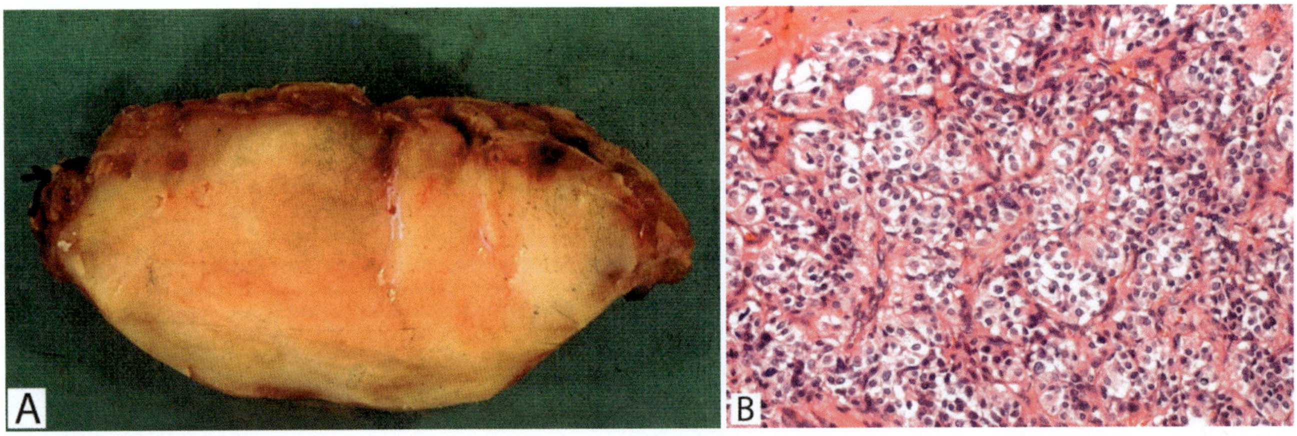

Fig 4.43 Thoracic paravertebral paraganglioma: (A) oval circumscribed yellowish mass in paravertebral sulcus; (B) typical organoid pattern of paraganglioma

Cervical Sympathetic Paragangliomas

Cervical paragangliomas are exceedingly rare tumors and too few cases have been reported to date to allow for accurate prognostication. There are fewer than 10 cases of cervical sympathetic paragangliomas reported as of 2004 (158). Most of the reported cases have been functionally active with excess catecholamine secretions and in some cases ipsilateral Horner's syndrome has been encountered .

References

1. Graham LS. Celiac accessory adrenal glands. Cancer 6:149, 1953.

2. O'Hare MJ, Monaghan P, Neville AM. The pathology of adrenocortical neoplasia: A correlated structural and functional approach to the diagnosis of malignant disease. Hum Pathol 10:137, 1979.

3. Harrison JH, Mahoney EM, Bennett AH. Tumors of the adrenal cortex. Cancer 32:1227, 1973.

4. Neville AM, O'Hare MJ. Histopathology of the human adrenal cortex. Clin Endocrinol Metab 14:791, 1985.

5. Conn JW, Knopf RF, Nesbit RM. Clinical characteristics of primary aldosteronism from an analysis of 145 cases. Am J Surg 107:159, 1964.

6. Third national cancer survey: Incidence data. National Cancer Institute Monograph 41:1975 DHEVX Publication No (NIH) 75.

7. Lewinsky BS, Grigor KM, Symington T et al. The clinical and pathological feature of "non-hormonal" adrenocortical tumors: Report of 20 new cases and review of the literature. Cancer 33:778, 1974.

8. Henley DJ, Van Herrden JA, Grant CS et al. Adrenal cortical carcinoma - a continuing challenge. Surgery 94:926, 1983.

9. King DR, Lack EE. Adrenal cortical carcinoma: A clinical and pathological study of 49 cases. Cancer 44:239, 1979.

10. Didolkar MS, Bescher RA, Elias EG et al. Natural history of adrenal cortical carcinoma: A clinicopathological study of 42 patients. Cancer 47:2153, 1981.

11. Nader S, Hickey RC, Sellin RV et al. Adrenal cortical carcinoma: A study of 77 cases. Cancer 52:707, 1983.

12. Slooten H van, Schakerg A, Smeenk D et al. Morphologic characteristics of benign and malignant adrenocortical tumors. Cancer 55:766, 1985.

13. MacFarlene DA. Cancer of the adrenal cortex: The natural history, prognosis and treatment in a study of Fifty five cases. Ann R Coll Surg Engl 23:155, 1958.

14. Cohn K, Gattesman L, Brennan A. Adrenal cortical carcinoma. Surgery 100:1170, 1986.

15. Tang CK, Gray GF. Adrenocortical neoplasm: Prognosis and morphology. Urology 5:691, 1975.

16. Hough AJ, Hollifield JW, Page DL et al. Prognostic factors in adrenal cortical tumors: A mathematical analysis of clinical and morphological data. Am J Clin Pathol 72:390, 1979.

17. Weiss LM. Comparative Histologic Study of 43 metastasizing and non-metastasizing adrenocortical tumors. Am J Surg Pathol 8:163, 1984.

18. Brabrand K, Soriele JA. Adrenal cortical carcinoma with invasion into inferior vena cava. Br J Surg 74:588, 1987.

19. Cagle PT, Hough A, Pyeher J et al. Comparison of adrenal cortical tumors in children and adults. Cancer 57:2235, 1986.

20 Weiss LM, Medeiros LJ, Vickery AL Pathological features of prognostic significance in adrenal cortical carcinoma Am J Surg Path 13:202, 1989

21 Aubert S, Wacrenier A, Leroy X, Devos P et al weiss system revisited: A clinico-pathological and immunohistochemical study of 49 Adrenal Cortical Tumors Am J Surg Pathol 26: 1612, 2002

22. Mattox JH, Phelan S. The evaluation of adult females with testosterone producing neoplasms of the adrenal cortex. Surg Gynecol Obstet 164:98, 1987.

23. Klein FA, Miller NL, Hodder RH. Flow cytometry in feminizing adrenocortical carcinoma. J Urol 134:933, 1985.

24. Hosaka Y, Rainwater LM, Grant CS et al. Adrenocortical carcinoma: Nuclear deoxyribonucleic acid ploidy studied by flow cytometry. Surgery 102:1027, 1987.

25. Sullivan M, Boileau M, Hogdes CE. Adrenal cortical carcinoma. J Urol 120:660, 1978.

26. Huvos AG, Hajdu SI, Brassfield RD et al. Adrenal cortical carcinoma: Clinicopathological study of 34 cases. Cancer 25:354, 1970.

27. Spain DM, Weinsaft P. Solitary adrenal cortical adenoma in elderly female: Frequency. Arch Pathol 78:231, 1964.

28. Hedeland H, Ostberg G, Hokfert B. On the Prevalence of adrenocortical adenomas in autopsy material in relation to hypertension and diabetes. Act Med Scand 184:211, 1968.

29. Copeland PM. The incidentally discovered adrenal mass. Ann Intern Med 98:940, 1983.

30. Abecassis M, McLaughlin MJ, Langer B et al. Serendipitous adrenal masses: Prevalence, significance and management. Am J Surg 149:783, 1985.

31. Prinz RA, Brooks MH, Churchill R et al. Incidental asymptomatic adrenal masses detected by computed tomographic scanning. JAMA 248:701, 1982.

32. Francis IR, Smid A, Gross MD et al. Adrenal masses in oncologic patients: Functional and morphologic evaluation. Radiology 166:353, 1988.

33. Kutz RL, Shikoda A. Diagnostic approach to incidental adrenal nodules in cancer patients: Results of a clinical, radiologic and fine needle aspiration study. Cancer 55:1995, 1985.

34. Orth DN, Little GW. Results of Treatment in 108 patients with Cushing's syndrome. New Engl J Med 285:243, 1971.

35. Gold EM. The Cushing's syndromes: Changing view of diagnosis and treatment. Ann Intern Med 90:829, 1979.

36. Lindsay JR, Lieman LK. Differential diagnosis and imaging in Cushing's syndrome. Endocrinol Metab Clin North Am 34(2) 385, 2005

37. Boggan JE, Tyrrell JB, Wilson CB. Transsphenoidal microsurgical management of Cushing's disease: Report of 100 cases. J Neurosurg 59:195, 1983.

38. Gruhn JG, Gould VE. The adrenal glands. In: Kissane JM(ed). Anderson's Pathology. 9th ed. St Louis: Mosby 1990, 1580.

39. Lacroix A, Bourdeau I. Bilateral Adrenal Cushing's Syndrome: Macronodular Adrenal Hyperplasia and Primary Pigmented Nodular Adrenocortical Disease. Endocrinol Metab Clin N Am 34:441, 2005

40. Azzopardi JG, Williams ED. Pathology of "nonendocrine" tumors associated Cushing's syndrome. Cancer 22:274, 1968.

41. Skrabeneck P, Powell D. Unifying concept of non-pituitary ACTH-secreting tumors: Evidence of common origin of neural crest tumors, carcinoids and oat cell carcinomas. Cancer 42:1663, 1978.

42. Singer W, Kovacs K, Ryan N et al. Ectopic ACTH syndrome: Clinico-pathological correlations. J Clin Pathol 31:591, 1978.

43. Jey RK, Can Herrden JA, Carpenter PC et al. Ectopic ACTH syndrome: Diagnostic and therapeutic aspects. Am J Surg 149:276, 1985.

44. Terzolo M, Bovio S, Reimondo S, et al. Subclinical Cushing's syndrome in Adrenal Incidentalomas. Endocrinol Metab Clin N Am 34:423, 2005

45. Reineke M. Subclinical Cushing's syndrome. Endocrinol Metab Clin N Am 29: 43, 2000

46. Bravo EL. Primary Aldosteronism. Urologic Clin North Am 16:481, 1989.

47. Page DL, DeLellis RA, Hough A. Tumors of the adrenal. In: Atlas of tumor pathology, ser 2, fascicle 23. Washington DC: AFIP, 1986.

48. Davis DA, Madeline NM. Spironolactone (aldoactone) bodies: Concentric lamellar formations in the adrenal cortices of patients treated with spironolactone. Am J Clin Pathol 54:22, 1970.

49. Cain DR, Van de Velde RL, Shapiro SJ. Spironolactone inclusions in an aldosteronoma. Am J Clin Pathol 61:412, 1974.

50. Gabrilove JL, Sharma DC, Wotiz HH et al. Feminizing adrenocortical tumors in the male: A review of 52 cases including a case report. Medicine 44:37, 1965.

51. Robinson MJ, Pardo V, Rywlin AM. Pigmented nodules (Blade adenomas) of the adrenal. An autopsy study of incidence, morphology and function. Hum Pathol 3:317, 1972.

52 Kameyama K, Takami H. Pigmented granules in functional black adenoma of the adrenal gland: A histochemical and ultrastructural study. Endocrine Pathol 10, 1999

53. Lack EE, Travis WD, Oertel JE. Adrenal cortical neoplasms. In: Lack EE (ed). Pathology of the Adrenal Glands. New York: Churchill Livingstone, 1990, 115.

54. Liou LS, Kay R. Adrenocortical carcinoma in children: Review and recent innovations. Urol Clin North Am 27:403, 2000

54A. Michalkiewicz E, Sandrini R, Fig.ueiredo B, et al. Clinical and Outcome Characteristics of Children With Adrenocortical Tumors: A Report From the International Pediatric Adrenocortical Tumor Registry. J Clin Pathol 2004; 22:838-845

55. Saracco S, Abramowsky C, et al. Spontaneously regressing adrenocortical carcinoma in a newborn. Cancer 62:507, 1988

56. Medeiros LJ, Weiss LM, Vickery AL. Epithelial lined (True) cyst of the adrenal gland: A case report. Hum Pathol 20:491, 1989.

57. Medeiros LJ, Lewandrowski KB, Vickery AL. Adrenal pseudocyst: A clinical and pathological Study of eight cases. Hum Pathol 20:660, 1989.

58. Vyberg M, Sestoff L. Combined Adrenal myelolipoma and adenoma associated with Cushing's Syndrome. Am J Clin Pathol 86:541, 1986.

59. Dieckman KP, Hamm B, Pickartz H et al. Adrenal myelolipoma: Clinical, radiologic and histologic features. Urologic 29:1, 1987.

60. Nobel MJ, Montague DK, Levine HS. Myelolipoma: An unusual surgical lesion of the adrenal gland. Cancer 49:952, 1982.

61. Boudreauz D, Waisman J, Skinner DG et al. Giant adrenal myelolipoma and testicular interstitial cell tumor in a man with congenital 21-hydroxylase deficiency. Am J Surg Pathol 3:109, 1979.

62. Guin GH, Gilbert EE, Jones B. Incidental neuroblastomas in infants. Am J Clin Pathol 51:126, 1969.

63. Turkel SB, Itabashi HH. The natural history of neuroblastic cells in the fetal adrenal gland. Am J Pathol 76:225, 1974.

64. Kushner BH, Gilbert G, Henson L. Familial neuroblastoma: Case reports, literature review and etiologic consideration. Cancer 57:1887, 1986.

65. Kaudson AG, Meadows AT. Developmental genetics of neuroblastoma. J Natl Cancer Inst 57:675, 1976.

66. Seeler RA, Israel JN, Royal JE et al. Ganglioneuroblastoma and fetal hydantoin-alcohol syndromes. Pediatrics 63:544, 1970.

67. Pendergrass TW. Letter: Fetal hydantoin syndrome and neuroblastoma. Lancet 2:150, 1976.

68. Dehner LP. Pediatric surgical pathology. 2nd ed. Baltimore: Williams & Wilkins, 560.

69. Rosen EM, Cassady JR, Frantz CN et al. Neuroblastoma: The joint centre for radiation therapy/Dana Farber Cancer Institute/ Children's Hospital experience. J Clin Oncol 2:719, 1984.

70. Weinblatt ME, Heisel MA, Siegel SE. Hypertension in children with neurogenic tumors. Pediatrics 71:947, 1983.

71. Jansen-Goemans A, Engelhardt J. Intractable diarrhea in a boy with vasoactive intestinal peptide producing ganglioneuroblastoma. Pediatrics 59:710, 1977.

72. LaBrosse EH, Comoy E, Bohnon C et al. Catecholamine metabolism in neuroblastoma. J Natl Cancer Inst 57:633, 1976.

73. Sawada T, Kidowaki T, Sakamoto I et al. Neuroblastoma mass screening for early detection and its prognosis. Cancer 53:2731, 1984.

74. Mills AE, Bird AR. Bone marrow changes in neuroblastoma. Pediatr Pathol 5:225, 1986.

75. Favret MC, Frappaz D, Maritaz O et al. Histological, cytological and immunological analyses are complimentary for the detection of neuroblastoma cells in bone marrow. Br J Cancer 54:637, 1986.

76. Tsokos M, Linnoila RI, Chandra RS et al. Neurone-specific enolase in the diagnosis of neuroblastomas and other small round cell tumors in children. Hum Pathol 15:575, 1984.

77. Gould VE. Synaptophysin: A new and promising pan-neuroendocrine marker. Arch Pathol Lab Med 111:791, 1987.

78. Angellati RH. Chromogranins and neuroendocrine secretion. Lab Invest 55:387, 1986.

79. Morales AR. Electron microscopy of human tumors. In: Fenoglio CM,Wolff M (eds). Progress in surgical pathology, New York: Masson Publishing, 1980: vol 1, 1980, 51.

80. Gaspar N, Hartman O, Munzer C, et al. Neuroblastoma in Adolescents. Cancer 98:349, 2003

81. Refaat M, Idris SZ, Blazkowsky LS. Case Report: An unusual case of Adrenal Neuroblastoma in Pregnancy. Oncologist 13:152, 2008

82 Kaye JA, Warhol MJ, Kretschmar C, et al. Neuroblastoma in Adults: Three Case Reports and a Review of the Literature. Cancer 58:1149, 1986

83. Folpe AL, Goldblum JR, Rubin BP, et al. Morphologic and Immunophenotypic Diversity in Ewing Family Tumors Am J Surg Pathol 29:1025, 2005

84. Angervall L, Enzinger FM. Extraskeletal neoplasm resembling Ewing's sarcoma Cancer 36:240, 1975

85. Jaffe R Santamaria M, Yunis, EJ et al. The neuroectodermal tumor of bone Am J Surg Pathol 8:885, 1984

86. de Alava E, Pardo J. Ewing Tumor: tumor biology and clinical application. Int J Surg Pathol 9:7, 2001.

87. Nilsson G, Wang M, Wejde J, et al. Detection of EWS/FLI-1 by immunostaining. An adjunctive tool in diagnosis of Ewing's sarcoma and primitive Neuroectodermal tumor on cytological samples and paraffin-embedded archival material Sarcoma 3:25, 1999

88 Folpe AL, Hill CE, Parham DM, et al. Immunohistochemical Detection of FLI-1 Protein Expression: A Study of 132 Round Cell Tumors With Emphasis on CD-99-Positive Mimics of Ewing's Sarcoma/Primitive Neuroectodermal Tumor. Am J Surg Pathol 24:1657, 2000.

89 Lewis TB, Coffin CM, Bernard PS. Differentiating Ewing's sarcoma from other round blue cell tumors using a RT_PCR translocation panel on formalin-fixed paraffin-embedded tissues Mod Pathol 20:397, 2007

90 Hiraga IN, Sawamura Y, Shinohe Y, Nagashima K. Alternative EWS-FLI-1 fusion gene and MIC2 expression in peripheral and central primitive neuroectodermal tumors. Neuropathy. 21:40, 2001

91. Argani P, Perez-Ordonez B, Xiao H, et al. Olfactory neuroblastoma is not related to the Ewing family of tumors: absence of EWS-FLI-1 gene fusion and MIC expression. Am J Surg Pathol 22:391, 1998

92. Beckwith JB, Martin RF. Observations on the histopathology of neuroblastomas. J Pediatr Surg 3:106, 1968.

93. Hughes M, Marsden HB, Palmer MK. Histologic Patterns of neuroblastoma related to prognosis and clinical staging. Cancer 34:1706, 1974.

94. McKinen J. Microscopic patterns as a guide to prognosis of neuroblastoma in childhood. Cancer 29:1637, 1972.

95. Gitlow SE, Dziedzic LB, Strauss L et al. Biochemical and histologic determinants in the prognosis of neuroblastoma. Cancer 32:898, 1973.

96. Shimada H, Ambros IM, Dehner LP, et al. The International Neuroblastoma Pathology Classification (The Shimada System) Cancer 86:364, 1999

97. Evans AE, D'Angio CJ, Randolph J. A proposed staging for children with neuroblastoma. Cancer 27:374, 1971.

97A Carlsen AU, Christensen IJ, Schroeder H et al Prognostic value of different staging systems in neuroblastoma and completeness of tumor excision Arch Dis Child 61:832, 1986.

98. Zeltzer PM, Maranges PJ, Evans AE et al. Serum neurone-specific enolase in children with neuroblastoma: Relationship to stage and disease course Cancer 57:1230, 1986.

99. Hann HL, Evans AE, Cohen IJ et al. Biologic differences between neuroblastoma stage IVS and IV: Measurement of serum ferritin and E-rosette inhibition in 30 children. New Engl J Med 305:425, 1981.

100. Evans AE, D'Angio GJ, Proport K et al. Prognostic factors in neuroblastoma. Cancer 59:1853, 1987.

101. Helman LJ, Cooper MJ, Cohen PS et al. Molecular biology of neuroblastoma and pheochromocytoma. In Lack EE (ed). Pathology of the Adrenal Glands. New York: Chruchill Livingstone, 1990, 311.

102. Krane NK. Clinically unsuspected pheochromocytomas experience at Henry Ford Hospital and a review of the literature. Arch Intern Med 146:54, 1986.

103. Medeiros LJ, Wolf BC, Balogh K et al. Adrenal pheochromocytoma: A Clinicopathological review of 60 cases. Hum Pathol 16:580, 1985.

104. Melicow MM. One hundred cases of pheochromocytoma (107 tumors) at the Columbia-Presbyterian Medical Centre, 1926-1976: A clinicopathological analysis. Cancer 40:1987, 1977.

105. Stackpole RH, Melicow MM, Uson AC. Pheochromocytoma in children: Report of 9 cases and review of the first 100 published cases with follow-up studies. J Pediatr 63:315, 1963.

106. Stringel G, Bin SH, Creighton R et al. Pheochromocytoma in children - an update. J Pediatr Surg 15:496, 1980.

107. Kaufman BH, Telander RI, Van Heerden JA et al. Pheochromocytoma in the pediatric age group: Current status. J Pediatr Surg 18:879, 1983.

108. Keiser HR, Doppman JL, Robertson CN et al. In Lack EE (ed). Pathology of the Adrenal Glands. New York: Churchill Livingstone, 1990, 237.

109. Steiner AL, Goodman AD, Powers SR. A study of a kindred with pheochromocytoma, medullary thyroid carcinoma, hyperparathyroidism and Cushing's disease. Multiple endocrine neoplasia, type 2. Medicine 47:371, 1968.

110. Gorlin RJ, Sedano HO, Vickers RA et al. Multiple mucosal neuromas, pheochromocytoma and medullary carcinoma of thyroid: A syndrome. Cancer 22:293, 1968.

111. Limnoila RF, Lack EE, Steinberg SM et al. Decreased expression of neuropeptides in malignant paragangliomas: An immunohistochemical study. Hum Pathol 19:41, 1988.

112. Modlin IM, Farndon JR, Shepherd A et al. Pheochromocytomas in 72 patients: Clinical and diagnostic features, treatment and long term results. Br J Surg 66:456, 1979.

113. Scott HW Jr., Gates JA, Nies AS et al. Pheochromocytoma: Present diagnosis and management. Ann Surg 183:587, 1976.

114. Van Heerden JA, Sheps SG, Hamberger B et al. Pheochromocytoma: Current status and changing trends. Surgery 91:367, 1982.

115. Montalbano FP, Baronofsky ID, Ball H. Hyperplasia of the adrenal medulla: A clinical entity. JAMA 182:144, 1962.

116. Rudy FR, Bates RD, Cimorelli AJ et al. Adrenal medullary hyperplasia: A clinicopathological study of 4 cases. Hum Pathol 11:650, 1980.

117. Carner JA, Sizemore GW, Tyce GM. Bilateral adrenal medullary hyperplasia in multiple endocrine neoplasia, type 2: The precursor of bilateral pheochromocytoma. Mayo Clin Proc 50:3, 1975.

118. DeLellis RA, Wolfe HJ, Gagel RF et al. Adrenal medullary hyperplasia: A morphological analysis in patients with familial medullary thyroid carcinoma. Am J Pathol 83:177, 1976.

119 Boissy C, Mainguene C, Di Pietro G, et al. Adrenal medullary hyperplasia: a rare etiology of arterial hypertension-report of a case. Ann Pathol 19:38, 1999

120 Stenger AM, Frilling A, Schroder S, et al.Sporadic unilateral adrenal medullary hyperplasia-a rare cause of hypertension Chirurg. 67:448, 1996

121 Young BC, Loke TK, Tse TW, et al. Sporadic bilateral adrenal medullary hyperplasia: apparent false positive MIBG scan and expected MRI findings. Euro J Radiol 36: 281, 2000

122 Kura N, Igarashi K, Sekine H. Asymptomatic adrenal medullary hyperplasia detected with intraoperative hypertension: a case report. Hinyokika Kyo. 51:321, 2005

123. ReMine WH, Chong GC, van Heerden JA, et al: Pheochromocytoma: Current management of pheochromocytoma. Ann Surg 179:740, 1974

124. van Heerden JA, Sheps SG, Hamberger b, et al: Pheochromocytoma: Current status and changing trends. Surgery91:367, 1982

125. Medeiros LHJ, Wolf BC, Balogh K, Federman M: Adrenal Pheochromocytoma: A clinico-pathologic review of 60 cases. Hum Pathol 16:580, 1985

126. Aguilo F, Tamayo N, Vazquez-Quintana E, et al: Pheochromocytoma: A 20 year experience at the University Hospital. PRHS 10:135, 1991

127. Samaan NA, Hickey RC, Shutts PE: Diagnosis, localization and management of pheochromocytoma: Pitfalls and follow up in 41 patients. Cancer 62:2451, 1988

128. Neumann H, Berger DP, Sigmund G, Blum U et al: Pheochromocytomas, Multiple Endocrine Neoplasia 2, and von Hippel-Lindau Disease. N Engl J Med 329:1531, 1993

129. Astuti D, Douglas F, Lennard TW, et al: Germline SDHD mutation in familial pheochromocytoma. Lancet;357:1181, 2001

130. Neumann HPH, Bausch B, McWhitney SR et al. Germ-line mutations in nonsyndromic pheochromocytoma. N Engl J Med 346:1459, 2002

131. Dluhy RG. Pheochromocytoma-death of an axiom. N Engl J Med 346:1486, 2002

132. Neumann HP, Pawlu C, Peczkowska M, et al. Distinct clinical features of paraganglioma syndromes associated with SDHB AND SDHD gene mutations. JAMA; 292:943, 2004

133. Martin R, Hockey A, Walpole I, Goldblatt J. Variable penetrance of familial pheochromocytoma associated with von Hipple Lindau gene mutation,S68W. Hum Mutat. 12:71, 1998

134. Friedrich CA. von Hippel Lindau Syndrome. A pleomorphic condition. Cancer 86(11 Suppl): 2478, 1999

135. Prowse AH, Webster AR, Richards FM, et al. Somatic inactivation of the VHL gene in Von Hippel Lindau disease tumors. Am J Hum Genet 60:765, 1997

136. Koch CA, Mauro D, Walther MM, et al. Pheochromocytoma in von Hippel-Lindau Disease: Distinct histopathological Phenotype Compared to Pheochromocytoma in Multiple Endocrine Neoplasia Type 2. Endocrine Pathology 13: 17, 2002

137. Wilson RA, Ibanez ML. A comparative study of 14 cases of familial and non-familial pheochromocytomas. Hum Pathol 9:181, 1978

138. Cance WG, Wells SA Jr. Multiple endocrine neoplasia type 2 a. Curr Probl Surg 22:8, 1985

139. Lips KJM, van der sluys Veer J, Struyvenberg A et al. Bilateral occurrence of pheochromocytoma in patients with the multiple endocrine neoplasia syndrome type 2 a (Sipple's syndrome) Am J Med 70:1051, 1981

140. Carney JA, Sizemore GW, Hayles AB. Multiple endocrine neoplasia, type 2 b. Pathobiol Annu 8:105, 1978

141. Eng C, Clay D, Schuffenecker I, et al. The relationship between specific RET proto-oncogene mutations and disease phenotype in multiple endocrine neoplasia type 2. International RET mutational consortium analysis. JAMA 276:1575, 1996

142. Riccardi VM.von Recklinghausen neurofibromatosis. N Engl J Med. 305:1617, 1981

143. Walther MM, Herring J, Enquist E, Keiser HR, Linehan WM. Von Recklinghausen's disease and pheochromocytomas. J Urol. 162: 1582, 1999

144. Erem C, Onder EH, Ukinc K et al. Neurofibromatosis type 1 associated with pheochromocytoma: a case and a review of the literature. J Endocrinol Invest. 30:59, 2007

145. Astuti D, Latif F, Hallol A, et al. Gene mutations in the succinate dehydrogenase subunit SDHB cause susceptibility to familial pheochromocytoma and to familial paraganglioma. Am J Human Genet 69:49, 2002

146. Bausch B, Borozdin W, Neumann HPH (For European-American Pheochromocytoma Study Group)Clinical and Genetic Characteristics of Patients with Neurofibromatosis Type 1 and Pheochromocytoma. N Engl J Med 354:2729, 2006

147. Melicow MM: One hundred cases of pheochromocytoma (107 tumors) at the Columbia-Presbyterian Medical Center 19266; A clinico-pathological analysis. Cancer 40:1987, 1977

dcha148. Hayes WS, Davidson AJ, Grimley PM, Hartman DS. Extra-adrenal retroperitoneal paragangliomas: Clinic, pathologic and CT findings. AJR 155:1247, 1990

149. Sclafani LM, Woodruff JM, Brennan MF. Extra-adrenal retroperitoneal paragangliomas: Natural history and response to treatment. Surgery 108:1124, 1990

150. Lack EE, Cubilla Al, Woodruff JM, Lieberman PH. Extra-adrenal paragangliomas of the retroperitomeum: A clinico-pathological study of 12 tumors. Am J Surg Pathol 4:10901`20, 1980

151. Grignon DJ, Ro JY, Mackay B, et al. Paraganglioma of the urinary bladder: Immunohistochemical, electron microscopic and DNA Flow Cytometry study. Hum Pathol. 22:1162, 1991

152. Leetsma JE, Price EB,Jr. Paraganglioma of urinary bladder. Cancer 28:1063, 1971

153. Kairi-Vassilatou E, Argeitis J, Nika H, et al. Malignant paraganglioma of urinary bladder in a 44 year old female: clinico-pathological and immunohistochemical study of a rare entity and literature review. Eur Gynaecol Oncol 28:149, 2007

154. Zhou M, Epstein JL, Young RH. Paraganglioma of the urinary bladder: a lesion that may be misdiagnosed as urothelial carcinoma in transurethral resection specimens. Am J Surg Pathol. 28:94. 2004

155. Gallivan MVE, Chun B, Rowden G, Lack EE. Intrathoracic paravertebral malignant paragangllioma s. Arch Path Lab Med 104:46, 1980

156. Odze R, Begin LR. Malignant paragangliomas of the posterior mediastinum. A case report and review of the literature. Cancer 64:564, 1990

157. Moran CA, Suster S, Fischback N, Koss MN. Mediastinal paragangliomas: A clinicopathological and immunohistochemical study of 16 cases. Cancer 72: 2358, 1993

158. Tischler AS, Komminoth P. Extra-adrenal sympathetic paraganglioma: Cervical, nand Urinary bladder. In RA, Lloyd RV, Heitz PU, Eng C (Eds). World Health Organization Classification of Tumors. Pathology and Genetics of tumors of Endocrine Organs, IARC Press, Lyon France 2004

Printed in Dunstable, United Kingdom

91223541R00076